Praise for
The Laser Vision Breakthrough

"It is rare that a book serves as a resource for both patient and practitioner, but *The Laser Vision Breakthrough* achieves both with its excellent blend of science and good, practical advice. With the explosion of information in refractive surgery, this book is a must for the patient who wants to truly understand the process and make a well-informed decision."

—J. James Thimons, O.D.

"[This book] provides all the information anyone considering laser surgery should know."

—Maria C. Scott, M.D.

"I have had the dual privilege of contributing to this book as well as knowing the authors. This is the most comprehensive study I have seen of what a patient must consider when choosing whether to have laser vision correction and which surgeon should perform it."

—Anthony J. Kameen, M.D.

"Researching the pros and cons of laser vision correction takes so much time. This book is a great shortcut—all the details and answers you want, but someone else did the work to find them!"

—Susan Daugherty,
freelance writer

"*The Laser Vision Breakthrough* is the ultimate source for anyone considering laser eye surgery. It puts the reader in charge by providing accurate, up-to-the-minute information, along with advice from the experts—doctors who have successfully treated thousands of patients. This book is a must-read for anyone who is hungry for information about the miracle eye surgery that has changed so many lives."

—Harry N. Snyder, O.D.

The Laser Vision Breakthrough

Everything You Need to Consider Before Making the Decision

Stephen Brint, M.D.

Dennis Kennedy, O.D.

Corinne Kuypers-Denlinger

PRIMA HEALTH
A Division of Prima Publishing
3000 Lava Ridge Court • Roseville, California 95661
(800) 632-8676 • www.primahealth.com

Illustration of the eye (page 46) by Gale Mueller

Library of Congress Cataloging-in-Publication Data
Brint, Stephen F.
   The laser vision breakthrough : everything you need to consider before making the decision/ Stephen Brint, Dennis Kennedy, Corinne Kuypers-Denlinger.
     p. cm.
   Includes index.
   ISBN 0-7615-2087-2
   1. LASIK (Eye Surgery)--popular works. I. Kennedy, Dennis, O.D.,
     II. Kuypers-Denlinger, Corinne. III. Title.
RE336.B75   2000
617.7 55—dc21

                                                    99-089458
                                                    CIP

00 01 02 03 04 05 HH 10 9 8 7 6 5 4 3 2 1
Printed in the United States of America

How to Order
Single copies may be ordered from Prima Publishing, 3000 Lava Ridge Court, Roseville, CA 95661; telephone (800) 632-8676. Quantity discounts are also available. On your letterhead, include information concerning the intended use of the books and the number of books you wish to purchase.

Visit us online at www.primahealth.com

*To Jere, for your unwavering support and for
believing in the possibilities; and to
Tim and Sam, we're glad you are sharing our journey.*

Dennis Kennedy, O.D.
October 22, 1942–February 20, 2000

When asked how Dr. Kennedy would be remembered, his partner, Randy Houdel, paused only briefly and said, "If I were to say just one thing about how I will remember Dennis, it is that he was a man of great passion."

All who knew him would agree. He was passionate about his family, about his office staff, and about his work, both treating patients and training doctors in refractive surgery follow-up care. Dr. Kennedy passed on to so many others the joy he experienced in helping people discover the wonder of a world seen through their own eyes.

He will be remembered for his many professional accomplishments and cherished for his kindness, his warmth, and his ready smile.

Contents

Acknowledgments

This book is a result of the efforts of many. Most of the words are mine, but the content was developed with the support of my co-authors, clinical advisers, and associates at TLC Laser Eye Centers, without whom this project could not have been completed. To everyone who supported me in this project, my heartfelt thanks, but particularly my thanks go to the following:

First, to the doctors who contributed their expertise to ensure that this effort resulted in the most comprehensive consumer guide to laser vision correction yet available. Many thanks to:

Co-Authors

Stephen F. Brint, M.D.—co-author, friend, and "cyber-pal" throughout the development of this project. From the earliest days of our association, Dr. Brint always has treated me as a colleague, despite my lack of a medical degree, for which I am most appreciative. While teaching me the language of refractive surgery, he also taught me about excellence and dedication. His contributions to refractive surgery have earned him an international reputation as a pioneer in the industry. It has been a real delight to work with Steve on this book and on earlier projects.

Dennis Kennedy, O.D.—co-author and supporter. Dr. Kennedy gave freely of his time and expertise as often as he was able while coping with serious illness, for which I am most appreciative. He has earned the respect and admiration of his staff and his colleagues around the country for his staff and his accomplishments and standards of excellence.

Clinical Advisers

David Eldrige, O.D.

Richard Phillips, O.D.

David Sullins, O.D.

Harry Snyder, O.D.

Jim Thimons, O.D.

Cynthia Wike, O.D.

Anthony Kameen, M.D.

Jeffery Machat, M.D.

Roy Rubinfeld, M.D.

Mark Whitten, M.D.

Many thanks also to the Executive Team with TLC Laser Eye Centers, who encouraged the TLC centers to share with me their patient stories and supported my efforts every step of the way. Particularly, thanks to Elias Vamvakas, founder and CEO, who shared his insights with me about the business of laser vision correction and what the future might be like. And to Jeffery Machat, M.D., founder and national co-medical director, who patiently answered every question when I'm sure he had more pressing work to do.

Special thanks to Gary Jonas, executive vice president with TLC, without whom this book would not have been possible. Gary brought me in to the Executive Management Team of 20/20 Laser Centers before either one of us could spell ophthalmologist. We learned that and so much more, as we watched an industry grow out of the dreams of many. From Gary I also learned about leadership, teamwork, and trust.

Thanks also to Linda VanGrack Snyder who was my TLC cheerleader, supplier of information, and "first-line" reader, and to her assistant, Stephanie Tew.

To Bill Leonard, thanks for your advice and your unfailing good cheer. To Janet Ward, who allowed me to walk around the TLC Rockville center like I belonged there, thanks for letting the staff take time to help me out. Thanks, of course, to the entire staff of TLC Rockville, who always said, "No, you're not in the way," when clearly I was.

The same heartfelt thanks to the staff of Whitten Laser Eye Associates, who gave generously of their time and expertise, particularly Mark Whitten, M.D. I watch you and wonder how you do what you do with such apparent ease. Thank you, Fran Cardone, for reading every word of the manuscript and making sure that the technical aspects were just right.

Thanks also to Anthony Kameen, M.D., who contributed many thoughts and insights that became part of this book, and to Roy Rubinfeld, M.D., who made me laugh even as he taught me some of the finer points about laser vision correction. And to Jim Thimons, O.D., who more than once reminded me of what laser vision correction is all about.

I appreciate, too, those who gave me friendship and encouragement along the way, including Marilyn Cohen, Lisan Collins, Coni Fisher, Karen Levy, Betsy Karmin, Pat Kane, and Rita Perry, who was always ready to pitch in with a helping hand, as was Dawn Flint, Dr. Kennedy's assistant. My sister, Deanna Kuypers-Romano, who read the manuscript from the point of view of a prospective patient and promised me that the book would educate, not intimidate, and Dori Stehlin, who helped me really understand why laser vision correction just isn't right for some people. And, of course, thanks to my family, my husband, Jere, and sons, Tim and Sam; I promise to spend weekends with you again.

Your efforts are greatly appreciated.

Preface

Right from the outset my co-authors and I want you to know that all three of us are laser vision correction advocates.

Stephen F. Brint, M.D., is an internationally renowned pioneer of refractive surgery and was the first to perform LASIK in the United States. He also has written two textbooks for physicians and has a thriving refractive surgery practice in New Orleans, Louisiana, and in Boca Raton, Florida. Dr. Brint also had his own vision corrected with LASIK, using the excimer laser in 1997.

Dennis Kennedy, O.D., co-managed laser vision correction patients with Jeffery Machat, M.D., founder and national co–medical director of TLC Laser Eye Centers, for nearly a decade. He frequently presented lectures at professional association meetings on the subject of patient co-management and building a refractive practice, and hosted educational seminars for audiences of his peers.

And I am a former vice president of professional relations and clinical affairs with TLC Laser Eye Centers. In 1994, I helped launch 20/20 Laser Centers in Bethesda, Maryland, and was a member of its executive management team until TLC acquired the company. I am also a former patient. I had my vision corrected with PRK using the excimer laser in 1995, in Toronto, Canada, before the excimer laser was approved in the United States.

We continue to have close ties with TLC Laser Eye Centers. Ms. Denlinger is a stockholder as was Dr. Kennedy. Dr. Brint has no financial interest in any laser vision company other than his private practice in New Orleans, and he performs surgery at TLC Boca Raton, Florida.

Having disclosed our relationship with TLC and our advocacy for laser vision correction, we also want you to know that we believe strongly that refractive surgery is not the right choice for some people for any number of reasons. We are not selling the procedure; we think the results speak for themselves and that you can make your own decision once given the facts. We have made every effort to present a balanced picture of the risks and benefits of this surgical procedure. This book will tell you what you need to know to take the next step in the process of deciding whether or not laser vision correction is right for you.

As you read this book and go through your decision-making process, remember that laser vision correction is a process, not a product. As is true with other elective medical procedures, there are doctors and facilities competing for your health-care dollar. Marketing medical treatments is a relatively recent phenomenon and providers are borrowing a "sell the sizzle, deliver the steak" advertising strategy from consumer-product companies. Don't believe everything you read or hear, good or bad. This is your decision to make and yours alone, in consultation with an experienced eye-care professional. Our advice is: See the best, we'll help you with the rest.

Good luck!

Introduction

In all our lives there are defining moments, moments when we know that our lives afterward will never be quite the same.

One such moment occurred for me in 1994 when I traveled to Canada accompanying a group of ophthalmologists and optometrists to learn about a device called the excimer laser. With this laser a surgeon could correct nearsightedness using a state-of-the-art treatment called photorefractive keratectomy (PRK), which was not yet available in the United States.

While there, I met a 35-year-old computer engineer from Texas who made the journey to Toronto to have his −8.00 diopters of myopia corrected. That he had 8 diopters of myopia means he was very nearsighted. Vision is measured in diopters. When reading a prescription for glasses or contacts, a minus before the number means the person is nearsighted, or has poor distance vision. A plus before the number means they are farsighted, or have trouble seeing things that are close. The higher the number, the more blurry a person's vision. Someone with 8 diopters of myopia can't see the big E at the top of the eye chart without corrective lenses.

I don't remember the man's name, but I remember that he was extremely bright and very knowledgeable. He told me that he had been reading about the excimer laser treatment for nearsightedness since the mid-1980s, had followed its development, and had been biding his time until the technique was perfected enough for him to undergo treatment.

I remember him as articulate and sure of himself; some might even describe him as "cocky" or "arrogant," but likable, too. He told me he had been wearing "coke bottle" glasses since childhood and he hated them because they were a hindrance when sailing or snorkeling, two activities for which he expressed great passion. And because his lenses were so thick, the glasses changed his appearance and made him feel less attractive. He had worn contact lenses off and on but suffered from dry eyes (a condition in which an insufficient amount of tears are produced to keep the eye moist) and always ended up wearing glasses again. Radial keratotomy (RK) wasn't an option for him, he said, because his prescription was too strong and too many cuts would be required to achieve good vision. His vision would probably only be partially corrected. He also worried about his long-term visual stability. So, he waited until the time was right for him.

During the course of our conversation, I asked him several times if he was nervous. No, he insisted; he had learned everything he needed to know; he was confident in the technology and content with his decision. His pacing and fidgeting belied his expressed lack of nervousness, but I barely knew the man so I took his word for his state of mind.

Along with the group of eye doctors who were there to observe, I watched this man undergo PRK. When it was over, I watched him sit up in the laser chair, look toward the clock on the far wall, and burst into tears. Not a teardrop or two, but an outpouring of emotions so powerful it silenced the room.

I knew at that moment, as did the doctors who were with me, that this procedure was miraculous. Not a miracle, mind you; miracles are spontaneous events occurring without apparent evolution, and refractive surgery has been a century in development. But miraculous, in that people who have lived most of their lives dependent on eyeglasses or contact lenses can learn in an instant what it is to have normal vision.

I also wanted to share the feeling of exultation that comes when you no longer have to rely on eyeglasses or contact lenses to see clearly. So on June 20, 1995, I had my vision corrected with the excimer laser. My vision wasn't nearly as bad as my engineer friend's, but my relatively low myopia was coupled with an astigmatism, so both my near and far vision were blurry. Because I had already reached the age when reading becomes a challenge, and I wasn't prepared to spend hours looking for misplaced reading glasses—at least not yet—I elected to have monovision. Monovision means that one eye is treated, usually the dominant eye, to achieve good distance vision and the other is left untreated or is undercorrected to achieve good close vision. Many people who wear contact lenses accomplish the same thing by wearing a lens in one eye that does not completely correct their myopia. (Monovision is discussed in chapter 5.)

In any case, nearly five years later my distance vision is 20/30. This means I can drive without corrective lenses, and I can still read most things without glasses, although reading small print in dim light is no longer possible and I do have reading glasses for those occasions. But for all other activities I am without glasses or contacts, and it is the very best gift I have ever given myself.

Two Primary Considerations

Since that time I've talked with thousands of prospective and postsurgery patients and watched hundreds of doctors perform the procedure. I've learned that there are just two things that anyone interested in this procedure absolutely must take into consideration. All the other things that are important for patients to know fall under the category of patient education, which is the purpose of this book, and informed consent, which is the process of learning from your doctor the risks and benefits of laser vision correction and signing a document that states you understand and accept those risks.

Here is what you must consider.

Extremely Personal Decision

The decision to have laser vision correction is extremely personal and should not be made lightly. You only have two eyes and you must have a thorough understanding of the benefits as well as the risks of the surgery before making a decision. You should not be swayed by advertisements or by what your family—even your spouse—friends, or coworkers tell you to do, nor should you have the procedure because "everyone is doing it." The decision is yours and yours alone; not even your doctor should talk you into it.

Conversely, you should not allow yourself to be talked out of it by someone who is ill-informed or has heard that the procedure is not a good one. Your doctor should guide you through the decision-making process based on his or her privileged knowledge of your unique condition.

When interviewing patients and their spouses for this book, I spoke with one couple from Maryland. He was an internist in private practice. His refractive error was −9.75 in one eye and −8.75 in the other. His eyes also had slight astigmatism. To put that in perspective, of all the people who need lenses for distance vision more than 98 percent are less nearsighted than that. His wife worked with him in his practice. Her vision was normal. He told me that he had read about laser vision correction in professional journals, but it seemed experimental. There didn't seem to be a lot of long-term data on which to base a decision. However, at some point in the last couple of years patients began to respond to his routine medical-history question, "Have you ever had surgery?" with "No. Oh, wait, yes. I did have that laser eye surgery."

That answer started to be given with remarkable frequency. He thought to himself, "If all of these patients are willing to have this procedure, maybe it is safe and effective." He conducted his own research study. He pulled information from the Internet, he spoke with colleagues in the medical profession, and he asked probing questions of all patients who told him that they had had laser vision correction.

After a few months, he decided that the time was right and the procedure was sufficiently perfected to be reasonably safe. His wife, on the other hand, was not so easily convinced. Their teenage son had undergone eye surgery to treat a medical condition and the experience had been traumatic for the entire family. Why, she wondered, would anyone voluntarily undergo surgery to fix something that can be corrected without surgery? Why tamper with an otherwise healthy eye?

Then her husband's eye doctor, Dr. Roy Rubinfeld, showed her how her husband saw without his lenses. He put lenses in front of her eyes that blurred her vision in much the same way her husband's vision was blurred normally. She realized that to be unable to see past your nose could be a life-compromising handicap. She gave him her blessing. He had the surgery, and after a second procedure to "fine-tune" his vision he now enjoys "normal" 20/20 vision.

Experience Matters

The other thing you must take into consideration when contemplating laser vision correction is that this is not a simple procedure. In the hands of an experienced surgeon the likelihood that you will achieve an excellent result is very high. But complications do occur and it's then you want to be certain that you are under the care of someone who has treated not a handful of patients but hundreds or thousands.

Dr. Jeffery Machat, founder and national co–medical director of TLC Laser Eye Centers, has performed nearly 20,000 laser vision correction procedures since he began practicing ophthalmic surgery in 1992. He estimates that minor complications occur in 1 percent of the patients he treats and major complications in 0.1 percent. (See chapter 7 for a discussion of risks and complications.) But he emphasizes to candidates that he cannot possibly know which patient will experience a complication. Furthermore, he might operate on thousands of patients for several months, with no complications at all, and then two patients in a row will have complications.

He points out that for a surgeon to experience a complication during the procedure is not a concern. The concern is whether the doctor will know what to do when the situation arises. Says Dr. Machat, "That's when you want a surgeon with lots of experience." He also cautions patients not to be persuaded by a doctor who tells you that he or she has never had a complication. Comments Dr. Machat: "Surgeons are human. They make mistakes. Complications happen. If doctors say they have never had a complication, they either don't do surgery, or they're lying."

Dr. Mark Whitten, a surgeon who has performed more than 15,000 refractive procedures, concurs. When having patients sign the informed consent prior to surgery, Dr. Whitten tells them that "the reason a risk or complication is in the informed consent document is because it has happened to someone. It may not have happened to very many people, but it has happened to someone. You could be that someone."

Then he adds, "If you live your life by statistics, then statistically speaking it is unlikely that it will happen to you; however, if it does, the probability increases to 100 percent. If you can't tolerate that level of risk, then you probably shouldn't have the procedure."

Dr. Anthony Kameen emphasizes to patients that if they have ever tried contact lenses, even once, they have accepted a level of risk of something bad happening to their eyes that far exceeds the risks associated with laser vision correction. Most patients are shocked when they hear this.

Every single patient heals differently. In addition, certain routine complications are easily managed if detected early, but they can turn into sight-compromising problems if neglected. For these reasons, you want to be treated postoperatively by a doctor who has seen hundreds or thousands of laser vision correction patients—one who is confident enough to know when to consult someone even more experienced than he or she is. You want to be treated by a doctor who is part of a patient-management team, one who has a vast network of available resources.

With those cautionary words, you can proceed with confidence to determine whether or not you are a good candidate for laser vision correction. The technology and the technique have been in development for a very long time. The vast majority of people who undergo the procedure achieve results that allow them to function without glasses or contact lenses for most tasks. Some still require thin glasses for such things as night driving, and anyone age 40 or over will probably need reading glasses after the procedure, unless they opt for monovision.

Always keep in mind that the decision is yours. This book is not written to "sell" you on laser vision correction; the procedure and the results are good enough to sell themselves. It is written to help guide you through the decision-making process. My co-authors and I will take you from a discussion of how the eye works and common vision problems, to how to know whether or not you are a good candidate. We'll walk you step-by-step through the preoperative examination, the procedure, and postprocedure care. We'll suggest questions you might want to ask of laser vision correction providers to help you find a doctor who is right for you.

We will tell you about the state-of-the-art of laser technology and what the future might hold for the very few among you who have prescriptions that are too strong to treat with available equipment. We'll even tackle tough questions about cost and insurance coverage. We'll answer the most commonly asked questions and the questions patients don't often ask but should.

And throughout, we will talk about people just like you who now experience the wonder of laser vision correction.

This book will help you make an educated decision about a procedure that can permanently improve your vision. It will guide you in making a decision that's right for you.

1

What Is Laser Vision Correction?

Laser vision correction is the commonly used, or "patient-friendly," term for two surgical procedures in which a device called the excimer laser is used to correct certain common vision problems. These vision problems, called refractive errors, are corrected with eyeglasses or contact lenses, and increasingly with surgery. The refractive errors are also known as nearsightedness (poor distance vision), farsightedness (excessive strain on the eye's focusing muscles, especially for near vision), and astigmatism (blurred and double vision, near and far). (To learn how the eye works and details about refractive errors, read chapter 3.)

Another common vision problem that almost always starts to bother people once they reach their 40s is called presbyopia. It's when your arms are too short to hold a book or magazine at a comfortable distance for reading. If you aren't there yet, the reference won't mean much. But if you are, you know what it's like to hold reading material farther and farther away from you in order to see print clearly. Eventually, you can't hold it far enough away and you have to get reading glasses. It happens to all of us, to a greater or lesser degree. Nearsighted people, however, can take their glasses off to read and in that way forestall the need for bifocals or reading glasses for some time.

Presbyopia results from a loss of focusing power, not from a refractive error. At present, the laser used to treat refractive errors cannot be used to treat presbyopia, but there are techniques doctors can use to correct your vision so that the need for reading glasses is delayed. And researchers also are working on lasers and other surgical techniques that will treat presbyopia.

Reshaping the Cornea

Using the computer-controlled excimer laser, a surgeon can reshape your cornea in such a way that your vision is corrected just as it would be if you wore contact lenses or glasses, except that the correction is permanent. This doesn't mean that your vision can't or won't change over time; it might. Many people become more myopic as they age; others become hyperopic.

The laser can't correct for naturally occurring, age-related, or future physiological changes. If you were destined to become more myopic or hyperopic over time, you almost certainly will after the procedure as well. It isn't possible to know now whether you will or you won't. Surgeons do factor in age when determining how to correct your vision, in anticipation of potential age-related changes. If your vision does change over time, the change may be so slight and may occur so gradually that you don't even notice it.

In simple terms, the laser transfers your current eyeglasses or contact lens prescription onto the surface of your eye. The reshaping is accomplished through a process called photoablation, whereby an intense, precisely controlled beam of ultraviolet laser light is used to stimulate the molecules of your cornea to the point where certain targeted molecules break and vaporize. Even more remarkable, tissue around and underneath the point of ablation is not affected because the wavelength of light generated by the excimer laser is on the cool end of the light spectrum and because the full energy of the beam is absorbed by 1 micron of tissue. One micron is equal to one-millionth of a meter. (See chapter 9 for a discussion of how lasers work.)

> *In simple terms, the laser transfers your current eyeglasses or contact lens prescription onto the surface of your eye.*

Vaporizing tissue may sound alarming, but you must realize that the laser removes only 0.25 microns of corneal tissue at a time, which is 1/500th of the thickness of a human hair. A human hair is about 125 microns thick. It would take 500 laser pulses to break through a human hair. The human cornea varies in thickness from about 500 to 600 microns. It would take 2,000 pulses for the laser beam to pass completely through the cornea. When using the laser to correct refractive errors, surgeons remove between 10 and 160 microns of tissue, always being mindful to preserve the cornea's strength by ensuring that sufficient tissue remains after refractive surgery.

When surgeons treat myopia (nearsightedness), where the cornea is too steep, tissue is removed from the center of the cornea to "flatten" the surface. When surgeons treat hyperopia (farsightedness), where the cornea is too flat, tissue is removed from the outside perimeter of the area of the cornea through which light passes—called the visual or optical zone, which includes the pupil and iris—to make the central portion of the cornea effectively "steeper." Removing tissue from the segment of corneal surface where the eye is unevenly shaped treats astigmatism. (For a discussion on how the eye works and how refractive errors change your vision, see chapter 3.)

Some people with very thin corneas should not have laser vision correction. Doctors may consider thin corneas to be a contraindication for surgery. Contraindication means a condition of a particular patient that may lead a doctor to conclude that surgery should not be performed on that person. A thorough eye examination prior to surgery is conducted to evaluate for corneal thickness, among other conditions that might rule out surgery. (See chapter 5.)

Achieving Desired Correction

When laser vision correction is performed, a technician programs the desired correction into the laser's computer with information provided by your surgeon and your eye doctor. The data, or refractive numbers, that will be entered into the computer are based on a variety of calculations.

Laser manufacturers supply software that includes an algorithm that tells the laser how many pulses are required to achieve a specific level of correction under ideal conditions; however, every laser is just a little different, as is every person. A patient's age contributes to the expected outcome; so do the temperature and humidity in the room where the laser is kept and the altitude of the community in which the laser operates, among other factors.

When calculating the level of correction needed to treat a specific patient, the surgeon uses the algorithm provided by the laser company, as well as his or her own adjustment factors, given the unique circumstances in which he or she operates and the characteristics of an individual patient. These adjustment factors are called nomograms.

Surgeons develop their nomograms over time by carefully monitoring patient results and adjusting accordingly the numbers they enter into the laser's computer for a targeted level of correction. Basically, they perfect their results for their particular laser and environment by a "trial and error" process of making adjustments after observing patient outcomes. This is one of the many reasons why it's a good idea to have your eyes treated by a surgeon who has done hundreds—or even better, thousands—of procedures rather than just a handful.

Based on the refractive numbers entered, the computer calculates how many laser pulses are necessary to achieve the desired level of correction. The surgeon determines precisely where on the surface of the cornea the laser beam is to be directed. As explained earlier, so exact is the control of the laser beam by the computer that tissue around and under the point of vaporization is untouched. Dr. Brint points out that "the goal is to greatly reduce a patient's refractive error. Many people who have their vision corrected with the laser no longer need to wear glasses or contact lenses at all. But some may wear corrective lenses for reading or for night driving."

Kerato Means Cornea

If you have heard about laser vision correction, then you probably have heard or seen written the two medical terms that describe the treatment of refractive errors with the excimer laser. They are *photorefractive keratectomy* (PRK) and *laser in situ keratomileusis* (LASIK). These are very technical terms for what amounts to the removal of minute amounts of tissue to change the way light is refracted, or bent, by the cornea.

Later in this chapter and elsewhere in the book, there will be references to various refractive surgical techniques. *Kerato* will be the common prefix; it is a Greek word that means "cornea." The suffix might be *tectomy,* which means "removal"; *totomy* refers to incisions; *plasty* means grafting or adding tissue; and *mileusis* meaning carving or chiseling. The preceding descriptive word or words refer to the technique or technology. *Photorefractive* means changing the refraction by the process of photoablation, or vaporization with light. *Laser in situ* refers to the application of the laser to the inner layer of the cornea, called the stroma.

You may also have come across the acronyms PTK, which stands for *phototherapeutic keratectomy*, and RK, or *radial keratotomy*. PTK refers to the use of the excimer laser to treat such eye conditions as corneal scarring or other abnormalities on the surface of the cornea that can interfere with vision. RK also is a refractive surgical procedure, but it does not involve the excimer laser.

In RK, surgeons use a diamond-tipped knife to cut incisions in a radial pattern to treat nearsightedness. The purpose, as in all surgical procedures to treat myopia, is to "flatten" the cornea and change the way light is bent or refracted. Studies suggest that RK is reasonably effective in people with lower degrees of myopia but that results are unpredictable in people with higher degrees of myopia. One data review, known as the PERK study, for Prospective Evaluation of Radial Keratotomy, also demonstrated that RK patients frequently experience a progressive drift toward hyperopia or farsightedness.

PRK and LASIK are the only two refractive surgical procedures that use the excimer laser to treat myopia, hyperopia, and astigmatism. Of the two, it's useful to think of LASIK as the next evolutionary step after PRK in the treatment of vision problems, although in fact they evolved concurrently.

PRK and LASIK Are Different Procedures

Although some doctors do continue to offer PRK to their patients as a vision correction alternative, most eye doctors presently performing refractive surgery recommend LASIK for most people. This is particularly true of doctors who have treated large numbers of patients. Doctors recommend LASIK because patients experience significantly less discomfort after the procedure and, generally speaking, achieve good visual results much more quickly than do PRK patients. In terms of ultimate visual outcome and the stability of those results, there doesn't seem to be a difference between patients treated with PRK and those treated with LASIK, except among the small group of the lens-wearing population that has very strong prescriptions. Data suggest that people with very high levels of myopia or hyperopia achieve better visual results with LASIK.

> *In terms of ultimate visual outcome and the stability of those results, there doesn't seem to be a difference between patients treated with PRK and those treated with LASIK, except among the small group of the lens-wearing population that has very strong prescriptions.*

The differences between the two procedures relate to the execution of the treatment with the laser, the amount of time it takes patients to achieve good visual results, and the potential for complications during and after surgery, all of which will be discussed in future chapters.

For purposes of describing the evolution of refractive surgery, the difference between the two procedures is that in PRK the surgeon first removes the outermost corneal cell layer, called the epithelium, and then applies the laser beam to the surface of the eye. Removal of the epithelium creates a corneal abrasion. If you have ever accidentally scratched the surface of your eye, then you know what it is to have a corneal abrasion. It can be quite painful; however, in PRK that discomfort is managed with anti-inflammatory eye drops and with the use of a low-powered contact lens that acts as a bandage over the wound until the epithelium grows back, usually within three to five days after treatment. Most patients experience mild to moderate discomfort, which usually diminishes with the use of over-the-counter medications such as Advil or Tylenol. Many also find that they are unusually sensitive to light, a condition called photophobia, and most people experience significant fluctuations in vision for the first few weeks. A few patients experience extreme discomfort and light sensitivity that lasts for more than a few days, and their vision takes months to stabilize.

> *In the hands of an experienced surgeon the entire procedure takes less than ten minutes.*

In LASIK, a thin layer of corneal tissue is first created with an instrument called a microkeratome. This layer, also called a flap or cap, is between 160 and 180 microns thick, slightly more than the thickness of a human hair, which as you remember is about 125 microns thick. The flap remains attached to the eye by a strip of tissue that forms a hinge, just as a metal hinge attaches a door to its frame. That flap is then lifted up off the surface of the eye and folded over, placing it out of the way of the laser beam. The laser beam is applied "in situ," within the cornea, on the part of the eye called the stroma. When the correct amount of laser energy has been delivered, the surgeon gently replaces the flap back into its original position. It remains in place through natural adhesion forces, without stitches.

In the hands of an experienced surgeon the entire procedure takes less than ten minutes. As a result, the technique has earned the somewhat irreverent name "flap and zap," hinting at an ease and efficiency that is in fact only true of highly experienced surgeons.

Both procedures result in the majority of patients—between 90 and 98 percent, depending on which laser-study statistics one reads—achieving visual acuity of 20/40 or better without glasses or contact lenses after one or more procedures. Visual acuity of 20/40 is good enough to legally drive a car in every state. Of course, there are a great many other factors besides visual acuity to consider when assessing whether a patient's visual outcome is acceptable or unacceptable, such as crispness of vision, contrast sensitivity, visual acuity in dim light, fluctuations in vision, and dry eyes. Each of these and other considerations will be discussed in a later chapter.

Suffice it to say that the visual outcome for most patients is excellent with PRK and with LASIK. However, LASIK is the more advanced technique. LASIK combines excimer laser technology with sophisticated surgical techniques developed over many years. Both PRK and LASIK are surgical treatments for refractive errors that have evolved over the past century.

Excimer Laser Development

It seems that all of a sudden we're hearing a lot about laser vision correction in news reports and human-interest stories in newspapers, in magazines, on television, and in advertising campaigns funded by providers of this treatment—both physicians and companies that own the laser facilities. And it seems as if everywhere we go, we meet someone who has just had, or is about to have, the procedure. As a result, we tend to think of this as something brand new.

That a laser is used to accomplish the treatment makes it seem not just new but somehow magical. Many doctors tell me that as soon as they mention the word *laser,* patients are ready to sign up for treatment without hearing a word about potential problems.

In fact, in the one-hundred-year-plus evolution of refractive surgery, laser vision correction is fairly recent, but it is not new. As you may remember from high school physics, the commonly used word *laser* actually is an acronym for "light amplification by stimulated emission of radiation." It was in 1960 that the first beam of laser light was emitted from a ruby crystal. Since then lasers have been put to use in medicine, in industry, and by the military.

Lasers have been used in ophthalmology since the early 1970s for the treatment of glaucoma, diabetic retinopathy, post–cataract surgery clouding, and retinal tears. In 1981 they became the subjects of study for the correction of refractive errors, when the excimer laser was shown to have an effect on corneal tissue. But even before that, in the early 1970s, researchers worked on using rare halides to produce laser action. In 1975 a researcher named Stuart Searles produced the first excimer laser action by bombarding a medium of xenon-bromide with an electron beam gun.

In 1983, Dr. Stephen Trokel, a research ophthalmologist at New York's Columbia-Presbyterian Medical Center, read of a physicist with the military who tested the excimer laser on animals to see what effect the beam had on tissue, including corneal tissue. Dr. Trokel also knew of the work of Dr. S. R. Srinivasan, and of a photochemist at IBM's Thomas J. Watson Research Center in Yorktown Heights, New York, who used the excimer laser to etch circuits into computer chips without melting the silicon from which they were made.

Trokel visited Srinivasan at the center and applied the excimer to cow eyes he had brought along. Later he visited optical engineer Charles Munnerlyn, who was working on a different type of excimer laser system with an electrical engineer named Terrance Clapham. In 1986 a company named Cooper Surgical began constructing Dr.

Munnerlyn's excimer laser, which was the first complete excimer system designed for potential use in the treatment of people. The Alcon Corporation later bought Cooper Surgical. The new entity, VISX Inc., became a public company and is now independent of Alcon.

Others were researching the use of excimer lasers in refractive surgery at the same time. They included engineers with Waltham, Massachusetts–based Summit Technology, and with Taunton Technologies, which bought VISX in 1990 and retained the VISX name.

It became a race to see who could reach the point of human clinical trials first. Before any medical device can be used on humans, it must go through a rigorous, carefully controlled investigative process called a clinical trial. It is part of the premarket approval process. The U.S. Food and Drug Administration (FDA) will not allow manufacturers of medical devices or products to sell them commercially until these items have been proven to be reasonably safe and effective. (See chapter 10 for a discussion of the FDA's approval process for medical products and devices.)

First Excimer Laser Procedure

Although other countries also hold manufacturers to high standards of performance for medical products and devices, physicians in other parts of the world have significantly more latitude in the use of experimental medical devices and thus are frequently ahead of the United States in applying new technology. In fact, the first clinical application of the excimer laser was by a German physician named Theo Seiler. In April 1985, Seiler used the excimer laser to create "cuts" in blind eyes, to determine the feasibility of astigmatic correction. Shortly afterward, Dr. Seiler performed the first excimer refractive surgery in a sighted eye, which had a malignant melanoma already scheduled for excision. He also ablated the first normally sighted eye in January 1987.

Six months later, in June 1987, Dr. Marguerite McDonald, an ophthalmologist working with Dr. Trokel from a laboratory at Louisiana State University, treated the first ten blind human eyes in anticipation of treating sighted eyes.

In 1988, Dr. McDonald was the first to correct a refractive error with PRK on a normally sighted eye during clinical trials for VISX.

In the spring of 1995, the FDA approved the Summit Excimed Excimer Laser for use in PTK, which is just for treating certain medical conditions.

In October 1995, the FDA approved the Summit Excimed Excimer Laser for use in PRK to treat refractive errors.

In March 1996, the FDA approved the VISX 20/20 Excimer Laser system for use in PRK to treat refractive errors.

Since then, the FDA has approved both lasers for treatment of higher degrees of myopia than they were originally approved for, as well as for treatment of hyperopia and astigmatism. Excimer lasers manufactured by four other companies, Nidek; Autonomous Technologies, a division of Summit Technology; Laser Vision Technologies; and most recently, Bausch & Lomb Surgical (which entered the laser manufacturing business with the purchase of Chiron Vision in 1997), also have received approval for use of their lasers in certain refractive procedures. Two other companies, Meditec and Novatec, also have excimer lasers in development. The differences between these lasers and what the future has in store, in terms of new techniques and new technologies, are discussed in chapter 7.

LASIK Achieves Century-Old Goal

Long before the excimer laser was considered a tool for vision correction, ophthalmologists were experimenting with various refractive surgical techniques. For all practical purposes, the excimer laser and refractive surgery developed in tandem. LASIK is the culmination of many researchers working collaboratively in both arenas, sharing data and building on each others' successes. LASIK is the realization of a century-old dream to permanently alter the human eye to enable people with refractive errors to achieve normal vision.

As far back as the mid-1800s there was an advertisement, presumably by an eye doctor, for an eyecup with a spring-mounted mallet that could flatten the cornea by striking it through the eyelid. The advertisement claimed that the device restored vision and rendered spectacles useless. (See chapter 8 for more on the marketing of laser vision correction.)

In 1898 a Dutch ophthalmologist, L. J. Lans, articulated the basic principles of keratotomy—use of incisions to reshape the cornea to change the way light is bent, or refracted, thereby redirecting images onto the retina rather than behind or in front of it.

In the 1930s a Japanese ophthalmologist, Sato, did some pioneering work in corneal incisions.

In 1949 Jose I. Barraquer, M.D., of Bogota, Colombia, began developing techniques for the surgical correction of refractive errors. He first attempted to make the cornea steeper by adding corneal tissue from a donor in a procedure called keratophakia. By 1963, Barraquer had invented a carpenter plane–like device called a microkeratome, which contains the blade used for cutting corneal tissue. This device was used to correct high levels of myopia in a procedure then called myopic keratomileusis (MKM) and to correct hyperopia, HKM, or hyperopic keratomileusis.

The microkeratome enabled Barraquer to cut a 300-micron layer of corneal tissue, which was removed, frozen, and then placed on a device called a cryolathe, which is used to shape contact lenses. After the tissue was reshaped on the lathe, it was thawed, placed on the eye, and sutured in place.

My co-author, Dr. Brint, was one of the first surgeons in the United States to perform MKM using the excimer laser rather than the cryolathe to shape the corneal cap. Dr. Stephen Slade, with whom I worked at TLC Laser Eye Centers, frequently regaled doctors at training sessions with stories of watching Dr. Brint carry the frozen corneal cap from the outpatient center where he performed surgery to his office across the street, where he had a Summit excimer laser. There he would reshape the corneal cap with the laser and then carry it to the center again to be sutured back onto the patient's eye.

Later modifications to MKM led to ALK, or automated lamellar keratomileusis. ALK is a procedure in which, first, a thin layer of cornea is used to create a cap, or flap; a second cut with the microkeratome is performed for the purpose of removing a small layer of corneal tissue, called the lenticle. Once the tissue has been removed, the cap or flap is replaced on the eye. Stitches were subsequently abandoned when surgeons realized that the corneal cap naturally adheres to the surface of the eye.

Originally, the microkeratome was a manual device. Today it is automated, driven by a motor and gears. The automated version was invented by Barraquer's associate, Luis Ruiz, M.D. Ruiz also refined the ALK technique, conceiving of keratomileusis in situ. With the motorized microkeratome, or automated corneal shaper, it became possible to cut and lift the corneal cap without removing it from the eye. Freezing, cryolathing, and suturing were no longer necessary. As the cap no longer was removed from the eye, there were fewer incidents of what were called "free" caps or lost corneal tissue. LK and ALK have more or less been abandoned in favor of LASIK, which is infinitely less risky and more precise.

Even as excimer laser technology was being refined, and laser manufacturers conducted clinical trials to demonstrate the safety and effectiveness of the device, ophthalmologists around the world were conceiving of ways to combine Ruiz's in situ keratomileusis with the precision of the excimer laser for removal of corneal tissue.

> *With the motorized microkeratome, or automated corneal shaper, it became possible to cut and lift the corneal cap without removing it from the eye.*

It was in 1990 that Italian ophthalmologist Lucio Buratto first combined the microkeratome and the excimer laser, using the microkeratome to create a flap and the laser to ablate tissue from the stroma (in situ).

Greek ophthalmologist Ioannis Pallikaris was the first to use the hinged flap technique and coined the term LASIK (laser in situ keratomileusis).

In June 1991, Dr. Stephen Brint performed the first LASIK procedure in the United States in his laser center in New Orleans, Louisiana. Dr. Brint was participating in clinical trials.

Other ophthalmologists who helped pioneer the field of excimer laser refractive surgery and keratomileusis include Ralph Berkeley, Daniel Durrie, Richard Lindstrom, Robert Maloney, George Waring, Fred Kremer, Mark Speaker, Lee Nordan, Jeffery Machat, and Howard Gimbel.

Others have experimented with techniques involving the grafting of donor tissue onto recipient corneas, called keratoplasties. There has been some success with every technique. But none have been as widely embraced as PRK and LASIK—not even radial keratotomy (RK), which has been around since the 1970s—because no other technique has proved to be as predictable in outcome or as manageable in terms of potentially sight-compromising complications. (See chapter 7 for a discussion of risks and complications.)

Evolution of Radial Keratotomy

Even as Barraquer, Ruiz, and others were developing surgical techniques involving the removal of corneal tissue, others were refining the incisional corneal surgical technique known as radial keratotomy. Although two Japanese ophthalmologists experimented with keratotomy to achieve refractive correction, the technique did not receive much attention until 1973 when a Russian doctor, Svyatoslav N. Fyodorov, was able to achieve results with some predictability.

Two stories have circulated as to how Dr. Fyodorov came to use radial keratotomy to correct refractive errors. One relates that a pilot who had injured his cornea with glass came to the doctor for treatment, and the doctor noted a significant improvement in the pilot's nearsightedness as the wounds healed. The other tells of a little boy who fell while riding his bicycle and broke his eyeglasses; shards of glass wounded his cornea. Subsequently, Dr. Fyodorov noted a marked change in the child's vision. Maybe both stories are true.

In any case, Dr. Fyodorov, in performing thousands of RK procedures, was able to reproduce results time and again with reasonable predictability. In 1978, American ophthalmologist Leo Bores introduced radial keratotomy to the United States. Since then, 300,000 RK procedures have been successfully performed. However, most eye doctors who recommend refractive surgery, recommend LASIK over PRK or RK for every level of correction. Those who continue to recommend PRK, for some patients with a minimal degree of myopia, choose PRK rather than RK because of its greater predictability.

RK is seldom, if ever, recommended for patients with moderate to high degrees of myopia because the greater the need for correction, the more incisions are required and the greater the possibility that the structural stability of the eye will be compromised. Furthermore, virtually all RK patients experience daily fluctuations in vision, becoming more nearsighted as the day wears on. In as many as 10 percent of such patients, the fluctuation is significant enough to require glasses for distance vision or for nighttime activities. Presbyopic patients who have had RK also experience difficulty with near vision in the early morning hours.

> *Most eye doctors who recommend refractive surgery, recommend LASIK over PRK or RK for every level of correction.*

Also, as revealed in the previously mentioned PERK study, nearly 43 percent of RK patients developed farsightedness months and sometimes years after undergoing the procedure. Patients with higher levels of correction experienced the most dramatic shifts. All RK patients experienced side effects immediately postsurgery, such as sensitivity to light and starbursts around bright lights at night. For most, but not all, RK patients these side effects diminish over time. The same side effects are fairly common among PRK and LASIK patients. However, excimer laser refractive patients seem to experience more rapid recovery, with LASIK patients generally recovering most quickly.

Vision Correction Alternatives

There are, of course, alternatives to laser vision correction, eyeglasses and contact lenses being the most widely used. Eyeglasses carry virtually no risk but don't necessarily give patients the best possible vision, particularly patients with extremely poor eyesight. The thicker the lenses, the more difficult it is to achieve good correction, and peripheral vision is compromised by the lenses and frames. Furthermore, patients who wear thick glasses also may have a problem at night with starbursting and glare around bright lights, as light bounces off the edges of their lenses.

Contact lenses most assuredly have risks associated with them. Contact lens patients also experience starbursting at night when light bounces off the edges of their lenses. People with dry eyes can quickly become extremely uncomfortable in contact lenses. And as optometrist Jim Thimons tells his patients, the "risk of infection is seven times greater with contact lenses than it is with laser vision correction. The risk of damage to the eye, to the surface of the eye, and to the shape of the globe is much greater with contact lenses than with laser vision correction." But he adds that with contact lenses there are none of the risks associated with surgery, which can have serious long-term ramifications.

The fact is that ever since spectacles were first invented in the 13th century, researchers have improved vision correction technology, and those who depend on optical aids have tried to lessen that dependence. Laser vision correction is the latest and best improvement to date, and one that likely will remain state of the art for another decade or more. To the question "Should I wait for something better to come along?" (which will be more thoroughly discussed in chapter 9), consider what the experts have to say.

Dr. Machat, for example, tells a delightful story of a patient he treated nearly seven years ago. "The man was moderately myopic (−4.0 diopters). Today, his visual acuity is 20/15 uncorrected. He had, and has, no problem with glare or halos. His vision couldn't be better. Yet when he stopped by to visit me a couple of years ago, he saw that I had a brand new laser with a few more bells and whistles than the laser with which I had treated his vision." The former patient asked Dr. Machat, "Is this laser better than the laser you used on me?" To which Dr. Machat responded, "Well, yes, it is." The man replied, "Gosh, I should have waited!"

It begs the question, Waited for what? Clear, sharp, uncorrected vision of 20/15 is just about as good as it gets. Dr. Mark Whitten had his vision corrected in 1994 before the laser was even approved in the United States. Traveling to Canada, treated on the "old" VISX 20/20, Dr. Whitten's vision was corrected from −5.0 diopters to 20/15. He tells patients, "I just don't think that if I had my vision corrected today with the next generation VISX laser, the SmoothScan, that my vision would be any better."

> *Improvements are ongoing, and, yes, the technology keeps getting better, but if you wait for the next best thing you are missing an opportunity to make your workload lighter and your recreation time more pleasurable right now.*

Whitten reminds them that "there always will be better technology and improved techniques down the road. But for people with no unusual circumstances, such as pupils that are very large or corneas that are very thin, there will not be a perceptible difference in their vision correction with yet-to-be available technology than can be achieved today."

Many doctors compare it to buying a computer, a compact disc player, or a television set.

Improvements are ongoing, and, yes, the technology keeps getting better, but if you wait for the next best thing you are missing an opportunity to make your workload lighter and your recreation time more pleasurable right now.

You might also want to ask yourself that question popularized by Jack Nicholson in the movie *As Good as It Gets*, "Suppose, this *is* as good as it gets?" And for most laser vision correction candidates, existing technology and a century-long history of refinement in refractive technique ensure that a skilled surgeon can now greatly reduce dependence on eyeglasses and contact lenses. For most of the lens-wearing population, the technology available today will achieve visual results that are as good as it gets.

2

Who Has Laser Vision Correction?

When I first was approached about writing a consumer guide to laser vision correction and subsequently contacted Stephen Brint, M.D., and Dennis Kennedy, O.D., about working with me on the book, we thought to ourselves, "How hard can this be?" After all, we had been part of the laser vision correction industry since before it was an industry—since before the Food and Drug Administration (FDA) approved the excimer laser for use in PRK, and before anyone knew for sure that laser vision correction would ever actually be a viable alternative to eyeglasses and contact lenses in the United States.

Furthermore, Dr. Stephen Brint had performed PRK and LASIK on human seeing eyes since 1991 as part of the FDA study. He was the first to perform LASIK in the United States. (It already started to become widely available in Europe, South America, Canada, and elsewhere.) For nearly a decade Dr. Kennedy had co-managed laser vision correction patients with Dr. Jeffery Machat, founder and national co-medical director of TLC Laser Eye Centers.

Not only that, Dr. Brint and I both had firsthand experience as patients. In June 1995, I traveled to Canada and had my vision corrected in my right (dominant) eye, leaving my left (nondominant) eye untreated to achieve monovision, which allows me to see distance with one eye and read with the other. (See chapter 4 for a discussion of monovision.)

By 1997, Dr. Brint had not only performed thousands of LASIK procedures but had also had it performed on his own myopic eyes by Dr. Stephen Slade.

Surely, we thought to ourselves, we have the expertise to write a consumer guide and we thoroughly understand the process patients go through in making a decision about having the procedure. Anyway, that's what we thought, until we started talking with patients and prospective patients.

No Such Thing As a Typical Patient

I spoke with patients who had had PRK in Canada before the excimer laser was approved in the United States. Dr. Brint spoke with his own patients, whom he had treated in studies here in the United States. Both groups are composed of people who might be called "early adopters." You know who they are; they always have the latest gadgets. They had cell phones before the rest of us knew what a cell phone was and VCRs when there was still a chance that Beta, not VHS, would be the dominant format.

Larry Baden, a director at the National Endowment for the Arts, is an early adopter. Having worn glasses since the age of ten to correct his 20/800 vision in his left eye and 20/1,000 in his right, he flew to Canada in 1995 at age 43. So pleased was he with the experience that he recounted his story for *Washingtonian* magazine's January 1996 issue. Five months after surgery his vision was 20/30 in the right eye and 20/20 in the left.

It was an early adopter who inspired the launch of 20/20 Laser Centers. Gary Jonas, co-founder and CEO of

20/20, now executive vice president with TLC, explains: "I first learned of PRK in 1992 when a friend's wife had PRK in Canada. Donna Citrin is an avid horsewoman. She grew tired of having dirt under her contacts, causing her eyes to burn and tear. Her ophthalmologist, Dr. Roy Rubinfeld, referred her to a doctor in Canada, Ray Stein, who was permanently correcting nearsightedness with a device called an excimer laser. Drs. Rubinfeld and Stein had gone through ophthalmology residency together at Pennsylvania's Wills Eye Hospital and had remained close friends. Donna returned sold on the procedure and sold on the idea that it was a great business opportunity. Her husband, Dr. Charles Citrin, agreed.

"A radiologist and entrepreneur, he already had launched a successful chain of MRI centers in the Washington, D.C., area, and he was convinced that he could achieve even greater success with excimer laser photorefractive keratectomy (PRK)." Dr. Citrin approached Gary Jonas and several others about starting a company. They did. And for the first eighteen months they were in business, they generated revenues by facilitating appointments and travel for other "early adopters." More than 500 people from the northeast made the trip during that period of time.

Dr. Brint, who could see the future of the excimer laser, paid $500,000 out of his pocket to purchase one of the first five excimer lasers in the United States in 1990.

Laser Vision Correction Is a Process, Not a Product

During the course of our research, we also spoke with patients who had only just that minute walked out of the laser suite after having LASIK, some of whom had considered laser vision correction for years. Like the engineer mentioned in the Introduction, many people seem to reach a point when they become convinced that the technology is sufficiently refined and the technique good enough to give them the confidence they need to make the decision. For some, it's a process that takes only weeks or months; for others, it can take years.

The decision can come in the wake of a crisis such as a lost contact just before a critical life event, a wedding, a major competition, or a professional presentation. Or maybe the decision is made after a moment of panic in which, without glasses, people can't locate their children at the community swimming pool. Sometimes, it's a matter of patients gathering enough information to feel certain that they make the right decision. In Dr. Brint's case, it was after seeing the excellent results and happiness in his own patients. He just woke up one day and asked himself, "Why am I wearing contact lenses?" In every case, it's a process, and one that cannot be hurried.

> *Many people seem to reach a point when they become convinced that the technology is sufficiently refined and the technique good enough to give them the confidence they need to make the decision.*
> *For some, it's a process that takes only weeks or months; for others, it can take years.*

We spoke with people whose myopia or hyperopia was low to moderate and to those with extremely high refractive errors. We talked to patients who went through the procedure with barely a hint of discomfort and those who months later were still attempting to achieve the best possible vision. And we spoke with prospective patients who had considered the procedure and decided it was not for them. Or who learned of the procedure through friends, family, or colleagues and, although they might have been good candidates for the procedure, quite simply were not interested. They are satisfied with wearing glasses. For some people, eyeglasses are a fashion statement, part of who they are, and ridding themselves of corrective lenses is not a priority.

Then, besides working with Drs. Brint and Kennedy and hearing their experiences, I talked to other doctors, lots of doctors, both ophthalmologists and optometrists. Some I knew from my tenure with 20/20 Laser Centers and with TLC and others I had never met but knew they had been involved with laser vision correction for a long time. I spoke with doctors who, like some patients and like Drs. Brint and Kennedy, were "early adopters" of the technology, and I spoke with some who agonized over the decision about whether or not to recommend refractive surgery to their patients.

I also read everything I could about how people experienced laser vision correction. I invited the TLC centers to mail, phone, or fax me the very best patient story they had. What we learned from the interviews, from all that reading, and from the first-person accounts so generously shared with us is that there is no such thing as a "typical" refractive surgery patient. There are commonly expressed reasons for having the procedure and frequently used words to describe the experience before, during, and after surgery. But every single patient is unique; every experience is one of a kind.

You've probably read stories on the Internet or in your local newspaper, or watched interviews of laser vision correction patients on television. Usually, but not always, the stories are of athletes, such as baseball pitching great Gregg Maddux and world-famous golfer, Tiger Woods; or entertainers, including Barry Manilow and Courtney Cox. Actor John Goodman chose Dr. Brint to correct his vision after stumbling around trying to read cue cards without contact lenses. Or maybe you've read that supermodel Cindy Crawford had laser vision correction, and almost certainly you've read some journalist's account. Lots of journalists have had laser vision correction.

But if you dig deeper, you'll find lots of stories about ordinary people leading ordinary lives, except that they took the extraordinary step of having their vision permanently corrected with a laser.

The Motivation

Some professionals, such as firefighters and police officers choose laser vision correction because the alternative can be hazardous to their health. Glasses can become foggy from sweat, rain, or smoke. If, while battling a blaze or engaged in some conflict, these people were to lose a contact or drop their glasses, they would put themselves and others in danger.

Maybe you've come across a feature story in your local newspaper about a group of firefighters or police officers who were treated all on the same day at the same center by the same doctor. It's sort of a civil servant appreciation day. Sometimes participants receive a small reduction in the cost of the procedure. A discount may clinch the decision, but safety is what motivates most people. Allen Owenby, for example, with the Henderson County, South Carolina, Sheriff's Department, explained to a reporter, "I'm having my vision corrected for safety. As law enforcement officers, there are times when we have to go into homes or businesses that have been broken into. When it's cold outside, my glasses fog up when I enter and this is a dangerous situation."

Anthony Brigidini, of the Washington, D.C., police force, concurs, telling a *Washington Post* reporter that long days in court and nights spent at crime scenes were made all the more difficult because he wore contact lenses, which dried up and clouded over after hours of wear. "You're going through a door looking for a guy wanted for murder, you don't want to worry about whether you can see," Brigidini says. And now, after laser vision correction, he can.

Lt. Brian Aylesworth, a firefighter with the Mount Laurel Fire Department, had Dr. Mark Blecher perform LASIK to correct his nearsightedness. His vision now is 20/20 in his right eye and 20/15 in his left. As he explained to a reporter with the *Central Record* in Medford, New Jersey, "You can't see much of anything anyhow in a fire, and it's worse having your glasses off to accommodate the mask and air pack. With 20/20 vision it's a little bit more of a comfort zone. A little sight is better than nothing. Now I can see during a fire without glasses."

There also are some truly compelling human-interest stories. For example, a young woman named Melissa Buck, at the age of 24, had her vision corrected with the excimer laser and could for the first time in her entire life see without the use of corrective lenses. Treated in Greenville, South Carolina, by Dr. Jonathan Woolfson, Melissa started wearing contact lenses at a very young age. She was in and out of contacts most of her young life, relying on eyeglasses when contacts became difficult or uncomfortable. She also endured two surgeries to correct for weak muscle tone that caused her eyes first to drift inward and later outward. Her uncorrected vision was 20/400, and her corrected vision was 20/60.

Already challenged by poor vision, Melissa developed ulcers on her eyelids that were aggravated by wearing contact lenses, which led to scarring on her cornea. She then began the odyssey to permanently correct her vision, coming ultimately to Dr. Woolfson. He explained that while he could correct her vision, it was very likely her visual acuity wouldn't be any better after the surgery than the 20/60 it was with contact lenses before surgery.

To Melissa, that was still better than the prospect of more scarring and eyesight that could get progressively worse as a result. She gave the go-ahead for surgery on the eye that was most urgently in need of treatment. To everyone's amazement, including Dr. Woolfson's, Melissa's vision in the treated eye ended up better than it was with contact lenses before surgery. Her visual acuity is 20/40 without corrective lenses, something no one thought would happen. (See chapter 3 for a description of visual acuity.)

Occasionally, there are romantic tales to tell, such as that of the woman whose fiancé proposed to her with the cooperation of the entire staff at the Mount Laurel, New Jersey, TLC center. Often, when a patient first sits up from the laser bed after surgery, the doctor or a technician asks that person to look at a distant clock, which, before surgery, the patient would not have been able to read without glasses. With this woman, the doctor asked if she could read a sign someone held in the distance. It read: "Dear Christine, will you marry me? Love, Pete." First she cried, then she said yes.

There are delightful accounts of husbands giving wives laser vision correction as a birthday or anniversary present. Sometimes they even perform the procedure themselves, as did Dr. Joseph Bacotti of Garden City, Long Island, and Dr. Roy Rubinfeld of Bethesda, Maryland. Or parents giving their children the gift of unimpeded vision. In Greenville, South Carolina, Alice Lundberg was so pleased with the results of her procedure, she paid for all four of her children to have laser vision correction. Former patient Harry Luke returned with a son and daughter in tow. They both had laser vision correction.

Dr. Brint recounts the story of a husband and wife from Tennessee who both had their eyes corrected by him, then paid the expenses for at least eight of their relatives to come down and enjoy the new vision that they experienced.

Athletes Jump at the Chance to Improve Their Vision

Until Tiger Woods had his myopia treated with the excimer laser by Dr. Mark Whitten and followed with a near record-breaking winning streak, pro golfer Fred Funk was as close as the laser vision correction business came to having a "poster child." His story has been told in *USA Today*, in *Sports Illustrated*, and in sports sections of major, and not so major, newspapers across America. As the Associated Press article relates the tale: "Fred Funk never envisioned a turnaround in his golf game. He simply wanted to regain the ability to read a bedside alarm clock without squinting. But two days after undergoing laser eye surgery, Funk found himself atop the leader board at the 1998 Kemper Open. He finished third.

"A month later, Funk broke a two-year victory drought, winning the Deposit Guaranty Golf Classic. Three months after that, Funk finished second at the Buick Challenge. By the time the 1998 season ended, Funk had carved out his first $1 million (U.S.) season in 10 years on the PGA tour."

Did laser vision correction turn his game around, or was it just a coincidence? "It sure hasn't hurt," said Funk. "I've played some awfully good golf since I had it done. It's certainly been a factor in my game getting better, but I don't know how much."

Why was he willing to risk his eyesight, without which his career as a golfer would be over? Funk told a reporter with *Sports Illustrated*, "I hated changing my contacts, cleaning them all the time. They distracted me when I putted, too. I always seemed to be putting through a smudge." Besides, he knew of other athletes who success-fully had their vision treated with the laser—Tom Kite, for one, who asserts that for him the big payoff is improved peripheral vision and not having to wipe lenses when play-ing in the rain. Other PGA tour golfers who have had LASIK include Rich Beem, who like Fred was treated by Dr.

Mark Whitten; Tom Byrum, treated by Dr. Harry Huang; Kenny Perry, whose surgery was done by Dr. Jeff Machat; and Mark Brooks, treated by Dr. Robert Lehman in Arlington, Texas. Women golfers also have taken the plunge, including Pearl Sinn (by Dr. Mark Whitten).

In fact, golfers seem particularly inclined to have LASIK. TLC Indiana Laser Center hosted a Pro Golfer day. Eleven Section professionals lined up to have Dr. Michael Orr and Dr. Kevin Waltz correct their vision.

Olympic gold-medal hurdle champion Derrick Adkins lost a contact just before an important jump to qualify for the Olympic team and decided: no more. It was time to have his vision permanently corrected. Olympic gold-medal swimmer Amy Van Dyken came to the same conclusion. After World Cup Grand Prix dual mogul champion and Olympic hopeful Michelle Roark lost her contact lens in the snow minutes before the moguls finals in Japan, she made a side trip to Denver, Colorado. There Dr. George Pardos ensured that she would never have trouble with lost lenses and discomfort from dry mountain air again, at least not because she was dependent on corrective lenses.

A growing list of professional racecar drivers have chosen LASIK over eyeglasses and contact lenses, including Billy Roe, Paul Gentalozzi, and Lonnie Rush. And pro ball players from every sport are getting in step, including baseball player Wade Boggs, football quarterback Troy Aikman, and basketball point guard Emanual Davis.

Journalists Tell All

It would be easy to conclude that it makes sense for some people to have laser vision correction but not others—not most of us. For example, it makes sense for professional athletes to have their vision permanently corrected; their livelihood depends on excellent vision, and they can afford it. Firefighters and police officers have the public's as well as their own safety to think about. Besides, most published accounts reveal that some special offer was made as an inducement to take the plunge. We understand why the Melissa Bucks of the world would choose laser vision correction. Her vision correction alternatives are limited and becoming more so.

> *It makes sense for professional athletes to have their vision permanently corrected; their livelihood depends on excellent vision, and they can afford it.*

But athletes, civil servants, and the visually handicapped aren't alone. Lots of "regular folks" decide to turn themselves over to skilled surgeons in anticipation of a life without lost contact lenses, midnight trips to the store for cleaning solution, broken glasses, or missed recreational or professional opportunities resulting from a dependence on corrective lenses.

Journalists seem particularly inclined to go "under the laser." Of course, that might be because it gives them the opportunity to write or broadcast first-person accounts of their own refractive surgery experience. Often it's their only opportunity to dramatize events in their own lives. And dramatize they do.

It's from this group that you will hear the microkeratome referred to as a "lawnmower-like device," a "glorified cheese slicer," and a "whirring electric scalpel." After reading some of these accounts, I'm surprised anyone would even consider laser vision correction.

One of the liveliest descriptions of the process was published in the March 1999 issue of *Elle* magazine. Wrote Jean Godfrey-June: "It's five or so minutes of extreme, extreme anxiety. People are operating on your eyes, and you're there watching it, full-on, with no mood-altering substance to blunt your heart-thumping panic. . . . But there's no pain at all. And it's five minutes (per eye; it can take up to ten, depending on your prescription): They prop open your eyes with a series of medieval-torture-looking devices, tape back your lashes, drop in various liquids (topical anesthetic, disinfectant), and flash a light or two at you . . . while the pressure is high, they slice the flap with the keratome (which I unfortunately envisioned as a razor blade, and, truth be told, did feel—not in a pain way, but in an uhnh-I-can-tell-something-is-going-on-way)."

Why did she have the procedure? "I'm blind as a bat and I don't wear my glasses. Vain. Ridiculous. Except that vain, to me, is about a person who finds her looks so fabulously irresistible that even a little flaw—say, a pair of glasses—constitutes a sort of unbearable aesthetic pollution. Glasses, on me, however, are something different: the straw that breaks the camel's back, the unwanted accessory that tips the scales from 'presentable' to 'homely.'" She made up her mind after a friend with the very same prescription as hers underwent the procedure.

Making the Decision

Lots of people do the same thing. Interested, but uncertain, they take a "wait and see" approach. Wait and see how many other people have refractive surgery without incident and with no loss of vision. Writes Terrence Loose in the magazine *Coast Orange County*, "After years of fumbling with contact lenses as an answer to my 20/500 vision (the big E on the eye chart is 20/400), I decided to give laser surgery a closer look . . . five friends of mine have undergone the operation in the past year—all of them were amazed. So I had good reason to be confident."

Although everything about his recovery was normal, this journalist admits to exaggerated fear of infection and of rubbing loose the corneal flap, resulting in high anxiety for him and his family. However, he concludes the article as follows: "With each day, though, my recovery is becoming more sure. And so is my eyesight, which is hovering around 20/25. I have even managed to travel entire blocks—without reading the landscape out loud, that is. My wife remains unconvinced, however. In fact, she's looking into the possibility that the laser went a little too deep and hit my brain."

> *Lots of "regular folks" decide to turn themselves over to skilled surgeons in anticipation of a life without lost contact lenses, midnight trips to the store for cleaning solution, broken glasses, or missed recreational or professional opportunities resulting from a dependence on corrective lenses.*

For local morning news anchor Eric Paulson in New Orleans, it was getting up at 3 A.M. and stumbling around without his contacts, trying to read the teleprompter, that brought him to Dr. Brint. In that experience he found a great TV news story: a first-person account of the LASIK procedure.

For Father Samuel Scott, it was a general lack of comfort with both eyeglasses and contacts that led him to make the decision to have laser vision correction. When wearing glasses, he found that he would take them off and on while celebrating mass, which was disruptive. He also is an avid sportsmen who enjoys weight-lifting, swimming, bicycling, and running, all made more challenging when depending on corrective lenses.

In a letter to the staff of TLC Big Sky (Montana), Walt Backer, a division engineer with Montana Power Company, writes of his decision-making process as follows: "I've worn glasses for about thirty-seven years and contacts for about thirty-one years. My eyes have progressively gotten more nearsighted and settled around −10.00 diopters in both eyes. The last four or five years I've worn gas permeable contacts. These have given me approximately eight to ten hours of wearing time. Without contacts or glasses, I could only see clearly a few inches in front of my face. With my contacts I can see 20/15.

"When radial keratotomy became available, I thought this might be an option to be free of glasses and contacts. When I found that after the first procedure I still wouldn't be able to see the big 'E' at the top of the eye chart, I decided to wait until something better came along. . . . I talked to many people who had LASIK. When I could not find anyone with a negative response to any of my questions, I decided this was truly an effective and proven procedure.

"I then started checking to see if this was the best buy for my money. . . . I did find another center out of state that performs the same procedure. Their cost was a little more than half the cost of TLC's. However, the excimer laser they used wasn't FDA-approved, and there were not enough people to talk to who had the procedure at that facility. I also realized there would be other costs such as airfare, hotel and meals, and additional cost if I needed an enhancement. Not only that, I didn't know where I could go if a complication arose. By going elsewhere, I could have saved about $1,500, but I chose TLC.

"Being an engineer, I didn't make the final decision to go ahead with the procedure until I read the book *The Excimer—Fundamentals and Clinical Use* [a text book for physicians, written by Harold Stein, M.D.; Raymond Stein, M.D.; and Albert Cheskes, M.D.]. Then I was convinced that I made the right choice." Today, Walt Backer continues to enjoy excellent vision and enthusiastically endorses the procedure.

Joan Reich went looking for a procedure that would reduce her dependence on eyeglasses and found, at the same time, a new career. By age 46 she had two almost-grown sons, a marriage that didn't survive some business losses, and an irrepressible desire to get out from behind her eyeglasses.

She asked her ophthalmologist about RK, but he was adamantly opposed, insisting that it weakened the cornea and that the results were not predictable. He told her that the excimer laser showed some promise, but it wasn't available in the United States. So she waited. While waiting, she learned of a start-up company called 20/20 Laser Centers that had offices in Bethesda, Maryland, where she lived.

I've also learned that however they come to the decision, patients describe the experience and its aftermath in much the same way.

She was also looking for a new career direction, and the idea of working for a company that would introduce the excimer laser treatment to the United States was appealing. So she contacted the company, was offered a job coordinating the activities of patients traveling to Canada to have the procedure, and has been with them ever since. But she didn't wait for the laser to be approved in the United States. As soon as she was able, she flew to Canada and had her vision corrected. Her recovery was challenging. She had PRK and her epithelium took much longer than average to heal. As a result, she had difficulty driving for a week or so and was in some discomfort. Yet she has never regretted her decision.

To decide on laser vision correction, not everyone needs to read about the physics of the laser and the physiology of the procedure or join a company that provides the service. But most do come to it only after careful consideration, and most are glad they did.

For many people like Terrence Loose, when the realization hits that they can now see without corrective lenses, it can be an eye-opening experience (pun intended). Laser vision correction is an experience like few others. Whatever their motivation, whether it's an inability to wear contact lenses comfortably, job- or hobby-related safety concerns, freedom from the hassles and the hardships sometimes caused by dependence on corrective lenses, or—let's face it—vanity, people come to the decision in their own time. But I've also learned that however they come to the decision, patients describe the experience and its aftermath in much the same way.

The Experience

Roger M. is a 50-something entrepreneur with energy to burn. Until March 1999, he had +6.00 diopters of hyperopia (farsightedness), which required that he wear three different pairs of glasses to achieve good vision: one for distance vision; one for mid-range vision, such as working at a computer terminal; and another for near vision. Needless to say, he was constantly looking for one pair of glasses or the other, never having the right ones at hand when he needed them. When he learned that the excimer laser had been approved for use in the treatment of hyperopia, he went to visit his ophthalmologist, Roy Rubinfeld.

I met Roger at TLC Rockville, where Dr. Roy Rubinfeld was about to perform a second procedure on one of his eyes in an attempt to fine-tune his reading vision. When asked how he was doing, Roger launched into nothing less than a dissertation on what an exhilarating process he was

involved in—an odyssey, he called it. Beyond being enthu-
siastic about the results of his first procedure, he was articulate in presenting his disappointment at not achieving
"perfect" vision the first time around, as well as his wonder
at being able to see anything at all without first picking up
a pair of glasses. Contacts were out of the question, as he
couldn't find a pair that did the job.

Miracle *is a word commonly*
used to describe the procedure and its results.
Others are **amazement, joy,** *and* **wonder.**

"You know," he said, "this whole process has been
delightful. And I must tell you, when I woke up the day
after my first surgery, I was prepared to worship at the doctor's feet for the rest of my days, that's how miraculous it
was to me that I could see. That lasted for a week or so.
Then I started to have some dramatic fluctuations in vision,
and I thought to myself, 'Well, the doctor has clay feet, after
all.' But when I visited him, he helped me understand that
with vision as bad as mine was, you have to expect the
process of restoration to take some time. I am prepared to
follow the process to its conclusion, whatever that is.
Whatever the final outcome, whether it's good vision without glasses or whether I end up wearing corrective lenses
for some activities, this is still truly a miracle."

Miracle is a word commonly used to describe the procedure and its results. Others are *amazement, joy,* and *wonder.*
Wrote one woman in a letter to the staff of TLC Rocky
Mountain, "After having been completely dependent on
glasses and contact lenses for the last forty years, it has
been extremely exciting to 'see' again."

From another woman patient to the staff of TLC Big Sky,
"What could be better than looking at the world through

rose-colored glasses? The answer is easy. Looking at the world through laser vision correction. No glasses required! Sounds corny, but there is really no way to make someone understand this life-changing event. For thirty-two years I've been constrained by some type of visual prosthesis. Now I have the freedom of seeing the alarm clock in the morning without pounding around for my glasses. I no longer have to buy shampoo and conditioner with different-colored tops. I can see my children come down the waterslide without making them wear hunter's orange to identify them. What new-found freedom! The procedure itself seemed so simple and pain-free, yet it is hard to call this 'nothing short of a miracle' procedure simple."

Every person who has refractive surgery has a moment when he or she fully realizes the enormity of what has happened. I call them "aha" moments. I had a few of those myself. The first came just days after I had PRK in Canada. I looked out the window of my house into the backyard and for the very first time in the four years I had lived there, I could see that there were daisies and roses planted in the garden. The second occurred during the summer months. I was at the community pool with my two boys, the older one an adventurous diver. I noticed from the end of the pool farthest from the diving board that there was a group of people, children, grown-ups, even lifeguards, all standing around the diving well, watching and cheering as someone executed another flawless dive. That someone was my son and for the very first time, without putting on my glasses, I could identify him from all the way across the pool by the features of his face rather than by the color of his bathing suit.

Other people report hearing a noise in the night, reaching for their glasses, and realizing they don't need them anymore. Some tell me that they continue the habit of pushing their glasses up their nose and find they have no glasses to push. Many people tell me that for months afterward, they prepare to remove their contact lenses before going to bed and suddenly remember they don't wear contact lenses anymore. Some even say they miss the ritual just a little, because it was their way of "shutting down" for the night. But they don't miss it enough to go back to wearing lenses.

Nearly everyone who has laser vision correction has an "aha" moment. Some are dramatic, some ordinary. Nearly everyone, but not everyone, because some people are not happy with their results; their vision is not now as good as it was before they had laser vision correction. You should know these stories, too. Optometrist Richard Phillips tells of a man, a marksman by avocation, who came to TLC Tri Cities to have his vision corrected. He had simultaneous bilateral surgery. The first procedure was uneventful and his vision in that eye is now 20/20. However, with the second eye there was a complication and two years later he still does not see as well as he did before the first of several procedures. He professes no regrets and believes the surgeon and the center staff are doing all they can, adding that he went into the procedure fully informed and prepared for the possibility of a complication; nonetheless, he can't be pleased.

Yet you should not make your decision based on others' experiences but, rather, on what you need in your life. And that decision should be an informed one, with full knowledge of the benefits of this procedure and its risks. To help with your decision-making process, you have this book. My co-authors, Stephen Brint, M.D., and Dennis Kennedy, O.D., and I have left nothing to your imagination.

3

Am I a Candidate for Laser Vision Correction?

People who are motivated to reduce their dependence on glasses or contacts lenses to improve their quality of life are the best candidates for laser vision correction. Sometimes career opportunities, the freedom to participate in leisure activities, and just not having to fool with glasses and contacts are the compelling factors. Anyone considering refractive surgery must first make certain he or she has no medical condition that would rule out refractive surgery.

Professional athletes and other active people, including swimmers, hikers, gardeners, skiers, skydivers, cyclists, and runners, are good candidates. Laser vision correction enables them to participate in such activities without worrying about lost contacts, lenses fogging up, or broken eyeglasses.

Firefighters and police officers are good candidates. For them, a dependence on lenses can become a life-threatening handicap. Entertainers, salespeople, and others for whom appearance affects opportunities, attitude, or self-confidence also increasingly choose laser vision correction. Or people who desire the greater convenience and freedom of not depending entirely on glasses and contact lenses to see.

People who are willing to make a commitment to participate in their own treatment and to adhere to the simple postprocedure follow-up schedules make the best candidates. As do people who are willing to understand and accept the responsibility of, and the small degree of risk associated with, laser vision correction for the opportunity to enjoy more normal vision.

However, perfectionists aren't always the best candidates. People who have a need to see perfectly all the time, and who see that way now with contact lenses, may not want to give them up. Says Dr. Brint, "There are no guarantees that laser vision correction will give you that same 'perfect' vision that you have with your contact lenses. Many people with contact lenses don't have 'perfect' vision, but it seems 'perfect' to them. Usually, laser vision correction allows people to see as well or better than they do with their soft or astigmatic (toric) contact lenses."

> *People who are willing to make a commitment to participate in their own treatment and to adhere to the simple postprocedure follow-up schedules make the best candidates.*

If you were his patient, optometrist Jim Thimons would tell you that the only way to ensure the sharpest, clearest vision is to wear rigid gas-permeable lenses (RGP). Says Dr. Thimons: "If that level of visual precision is important to you and you are comfortable wearing RGPs for long periods of time, then laser vision correction might not be right for you at this point. However, you might reconsider surgery when you reach the point where you can no longer wear contacts for the length of time you need and want to.

"On the other hand," he adds, "if you have switched from RGPs to soft lenses, to extended-wear lenses, and then to daily wear, and if you also have multiple pairs of glasses, none of which seem quite right, it is probable that laser vision correction will give you vision that you can be comfortable with all the time."

People who are completely intolerant of risk are poor candidates. A friend of mine, Dori Stehlin, would seem to be an ideal candidate, from a clinical point of view. She is moderately myopic and has moderate astigmatism. She's in excellent health. She successfully wore contact lenses from the age of 14 until her mid-30s, when she became contact lens–intolerant, meaning she was unable to comfortably wear contacts for more than thirty minutes or so. Originally, she wore hard lenses; later she considered soft lenses but found that because of her astigmatism, she would not be able to wear them successfully.

Consequently, she now is completely dependent on eyeglasses. It isn't for lack of awareness about alternatives that she remains in glasses. As the former editor of *FDA Consumer* magazine she has assigned writers to cover the topic of excimer laser surgery and has edited their work, so she is certainly well informed. Since having the procedure myself and working in the industry, I've asked her more than once why she doesn't have laser vision correction. Her reply is always the same. "For me, any risk is too great a risk for a surgery that is not lifesaving. I wouldn't have cosmetic surgery, and I won't have my vision corrected with a laser."

On the other hand, anyone who believes that "those things mentioned in the informed consent document could never happen to me" are also people who should not have the procedure. As ophthalmologist Mark Whitten tells his patients, "That a complication is written into the informed consent document means it happened to someone, somewhere, sometime. You could be that someone."

People who have not taken the time to become educated about the procedure, the surgical process, and the postoperative recovery also make poor laser vision correction candidates because they are not as well-equipped to participate in the decision-making process, in their treatment, or in the necessary follow-up care. The more you know, the better you are able to make an informed decision as to whether laser vision correction is right for you.

The very first things you should know are how the eye works, what kind of vision problems people commonly experience, and how these are measured. This will help you to understand how the laser corrects vision problems. It also is important that you know about various contraindications, or conditions a person could have that would rule out laser vision correction. These will be discussed later in this chapter and in chapter 5.

Even people who are good candidates, from a clinical point of view—in other words, there is no optical or medical condition preventing them from having refractive surgery—may not be good candidates because they don't have the right "personality profile." Included in this group are people who will not be satisfied with anything less than absolute perfection.

Patients who decide to have laser vision correction because they absolutely have to throw away their lenses should reconsider surgery. No one can promise that you will never wear lenses again for certain tasks.

Optometrist Harry Snyder has practiced in the northern Virginia area for more than twenty years and was among the early group of optometrists to recommend refractive surgery to patients as an alternative to contact lenses or eyeglasses. Although he believes that refractive surgery is an excellent choice for many patients, he also will tell you that "Every eye doctor has treated patients whose examination takes an exceptionally long time because they agonize over the question 'Which one is better, one or two?' They struggle to try to see the 20/10 line because they take pride in their perfect vision.

"These people," says Dr. Snyder, "are people you don't want to encourage to have laser vision correction, because they will never be happy no matter how good their vision. Every little fluctuation in vision, anything less than their perception of perfect, will be a disappointment."

Patients who decide to have laser vision correction because they absolutely have to throw away their lenses should reconsider surgery. No one can promise that you will never wear lenses again for certain tasks, such as reading or night driving.

How the Eye Works

But first, here is a primer on how the eye works. As you probably remember from middle-school science classes and have probably read in one of the hundreds of brochures available about laser vision correction in print and on the Internet, the eye works something like a camera. Even though we use the analogy here, it's important for readers to appreciate that the eye is infinitely more complex than a camera and that all parts of the eye must operate optimally to achieve the best possible vision.

Sight is possible because everything that has mass reflects light. Light reflected off objects passes through our eyes until it reaches the retina, which is composed of ten layers of various tissues, including nerve cells, pigment cells, and blood vessels. One of the deepest layers contains light-sensitive cells called rods and cones. Rods are sensitive to black and white and are mostly used in dim light. Cones are sensitive to color and function best in bright light. The retina converts light into electrical impulses that are transmitted through the optic nerve to the brain, which translates those impulses into images. It's important to remember that although sight occurs in the eye, vision actually occurs in the occipital (rear) lobes of the brain.

Simple, yes? Not really.

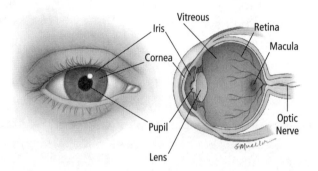

The parts of the eye.

Optical Gateways

For light to reach the retina, it must pass through a number of "optical gateways," components of the eye that have the potential to affect good vision.

Tear Film is a water, oil, and protein layer that makes the surface of the eye smooth. It has less thickness than a single cell but is crucial to vision, as it picks up light rays and bends them so that they enter the eye at an angle. Patients who suffer from dry eyes either lack a tear film or it has dried out. Sometimes the condition is chronic, sometimes temporary as a result of environmental factors.

The *cornea* is the outer surface of the eye and is a transparent "window to the world" through which light travels as it enters the eye. It is like the glass that covers the camera lens. The cornea provides 70 percent of the eye's refractive, or focusing, power.

The *pupil* is the opening in the iris (the colored part of your eye) in the middle of your eye, which seems to expand and contract as your eye adjusts to the amount of light passing through it. The pupil is like the hole in the middle of a camera's aperture, which gets bigger and smaller as the photographer adjusts the camera's focus.

The *iris* is the round, pigmented membrane surrounding the pupil, which has muscles to adjust the size of the pupil. The iris functions like a camera's aperture.

The *aqueous humor* is the fluid that fills the areas called the anterior and posterior chambers, both of which are between the cornea and the crystalline lens.

The *crystalline lens,* which lies behind the iris, is soft and flexible, at least until late middle age, and can redirect the angle at which light continues its journey through the eye. Although the cornea cannot change its focus or angle of refraction, the lens can adjust its power. This focusing process is called accommodation. Focusing muscles surrounding the lens contract to make the lens thick in the center to facilitate near vision and relax to make it thinner to improve distance vision.

As we age, our ability to accommodate for near objects diminishes and we become presbyopic. Then things at very close range are blurry. That's when we keep extending our arm farther and farther to read until we run out of arm, give up, and get reading glasses. Optometrist Richard Phillips describes one 70-year-old patient who had near perfect distance vision and claimed to not need glasses for reading. When Dr. Phillips asked him how he read the newspaper, the patient explained, "Oh, I put the paper on the floor and stand on a chair."

It is in the crystalline lens that cataracts form. Surgery is often required to remove the clouded lens and to implant a new lens made of a special kind of plastic. Generally speaking, cataracts are a problem for older people, although it is possible to develop cataracts at any time. Many of today's refractive surgeons refined their surgical skills over many years of treating patients with cataracts by removing and replacing the crystalline lens.

The *vitreous humor* is a very thick, gel-like fluid that fills the main cavity of the eye.

The *retina* is composed of ten layers of cells at the back of the eye and acts sort of like camera film, in that it is the receptor of the light from which images develop. The retina converts light into electrical impulses that are passed to the brain through the optic nerve.

Perfect Vision Is Rare

When all elements of the eye work perfectly together, vision is crisp and colors are sharp. Clarity of vision is called visual acuity and is expressed in numbers determined by a measurement from the Snellen Chart, named for its originator, Hermann Snellen. Anyone who wears corrective lenses has seen the Snellen Chart. It's the poster or projection with the big E at the top and random letters of decreasing size stacked in a sort of pyramid shape.

The standard against which visual acuity is measured is expressed as 20/20, which means a person with "normal" vision can see the 20/20 line clearly from 20 feet. A person with 20/100 vision would have to stand at 20 feet to see what a person with "normal" vision can see at 100 feet. Someone with visual acuity of 20/200 would have to stand at 20 feet to see what a person with "normal" vision can see at 200 feet, and so on. Someone with visual acuity of 20/400 probably can barely see the big E at the top of the chart.

Here's another way to think about it. Dr. Phillips explains to patients that "20/20 means you can see at 20 feet what you ought to be able to see at 20 feet. It's possible to have visual acuity of 20/15, which means that you can see at 20 feet what you should have to take five foot-long steps forward to see. Theoretically, you could get to 20/1, meaning you can see at 20 feet what a normally sighted person has to stand at one foot away to see clearly." Of course, Dr. Phillips has never examined a patient with 20/1 visual acuity. He's seen lots of 20/15s and even a few 20/10s, mostly pilots and baseball players who have to

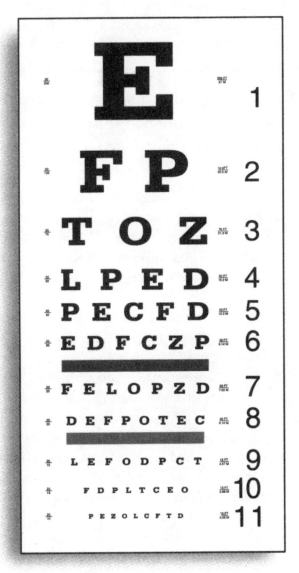

The Snellen Chart

have "eagle eyes" to make a quick judgment about where a ball traveling at speeds over 120 miles per hour might fall. That might be as close to perfect as anyone can get.

Much of the available literature about laser vision correction emphatically makes the point that most people who have the procedure achieve visual acuity of 20/40 or better. You now know this means that a person with 20/40 vision can see at 20 feet what a normally sighted person can see at 40 feet. In every state, visual acuity of 20/40 is considered good enough to drive a car without corrective lenses.

> *Only four people out of ten have natural visual acuity of 20/20. The rest of us have vision problems to a greater or lesser degree.*

It's also important to understand that having visual acuity of 20/20 does not necessarily mean your vision is perfect. Lots of people can read the 20/20 line on the Snellen Chart and probably don't depend on corrective lenses, but they still have what they consider less than perfect vision. They might be unusually sensitive to light, which makes vision in bright daylight more difficult. They might have dry eyes, which can cause vision to fluctuate during the day, depending upon how moist the cornea is as a result of their environment or their physical condition. Forced-air heat and air conditioning, for example, cause rooms to become drier, which can affect vision. Fatigue also causes fluctuations in vision. People with visual acuity of 20/20 might still have reduced contrast sensitivity, which, for example, might cause them to have difficulty at night reading street signs that are in muted colors.

Conversely, many people have 20/25 or even 20/40 best vision. To them, this is "perfect" because, for whatever medical reason, this is the only vision they have ever known.

For optimum visual acuity, the light that passes through these optical gateways must come to a point on a tiny spot on the retina called the macula. This spot is just 1/20 of an inch in diameter. Given that light has to travel through the tear film, cornea, aqueous humor, pupil, crystalline lens, and vitreous humor, and end up at a single point on the retina, it's a wonder that any of us have good natural vision.

And, in fact, the majority of us do not have perfect vision. Only four people out of ten have natural visual acuity of 20/20. The rest of us have vision problems to a greater or lesser degree. Light either falls in front of the retina, making us nearsighted; it falls behind the retina, making us farsighted; or our cornea is irregularly shaped, causing light to fall in two different focal points, making us

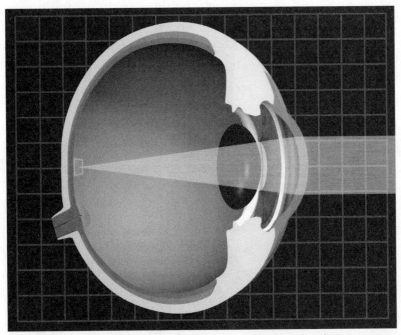

When light rays fall properly on the retina, as in this illustration, unaided vision is sharp and clear. A person with good normal vision has visual acuity of 20/20.

astigmatic. And, of course, there are those of us over 40 whose crystalline lenses are less able to accommodate for distance and near vision, making us presbyopic, which is Latin for "old sight."

Common Vision Problems

If you are one of the six out of ten people with a refractive error that is significant enough to require corrective lenses for some or all tasks, you might be nearsighted (myopic), farsighted (hyperopic), astigmatic, or presbyopic. Greater than 50 percent of people with myopia or hyperopia also have astigmatism. Each is described further on.

Myopia

Myopia (nearsightedness) results in poor distance vision because, as Dr. Phillips explains to patients, "If you are nearsighted, your eye is too long, too strong, or too highly curved, giving it too much focusing power." Focusing power refers to the ability of the cornea and the crystalline lens to refract, or bend, light so that the rays fall properly on the retina. Much of the literature on laser vision correction describes myopia as a condition caused by a cornea that is too curved, which slightly oversimplifies the condition.

The cornea may be too curved, giving it too much focusing power and thereby causing light to fall in front of the retina. However, myopia also results when the cornea

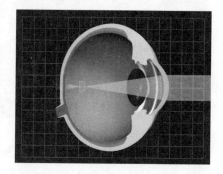

An eye that is too long, or that has a cornea with too much of a curve, has too much focusing power and is said to be myopic. People with myopia have difficulty with distance vision. Myopia is expressed in negative numbers because corrective lenses have to take away focusing power.

has proper focusing power but the eye is longer than a "normal" eye. Then, too, light will fall in front of, rather than on, the retina.

To compensate for nearsightedness, doctors prescribe lenses that reduce the eyes' focusing power. The lenses take away power, hence the minus (−) in front of an eyeglasses or contact lens prescription for myopia.

Hyperopia

Hyperopia (farsightedness) refers to the opposite problem. The cornea and crystalline lens working together don't have enough focusing power to ensure that light falls properly on the retina. Instead, rays come to a point or dissipate behind the retina. Again, this can be caused by an eye that is too short for the amount of focusing power provided by the cornea and the crystalline lens or a cornea that is too flat or weak. To compensate for farsightedness, doctors prescribe lenses that add focusing power, hence the plus (+) in front of a prescription of a patient with hyperopia.

The eye wants to see. So, younger people with hyperopia have a slight advantage over young nearsighted individuals because their eyes are able to work and bring into focus distant objects and work even a little harder to bring near objects into focus to accommodate for the lack of a focal point. However, as hyperopes age, they lose that ability to accommodate and are then at a greater disadvantage than myopes are. For example, nearsighted

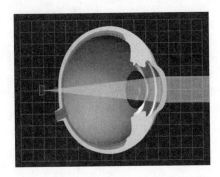

An eye that is too short or that has a cornea with not enough of a curve is said to be hyperopic. People with hyperopia have difficulty with near vision. Hyperopia is expressed in plus (+) numbers because corrective lenses add focusing power.

people often can remove their distance lenses to bring near things into focus. You've probably seen many people lift their glasses to read a menu or the fine print on package labels at the supermarket. However, with hyperopia the opposite is true. The greater the degree of farsightedness, the more difficult it is to see distant objects clearly, and close objects can become nearly impossible to see without glasses.

Astigmatism

This is also true for people with moderate to high degrees of astigmatism, although for a different reason. Derived from Latin, *astigmatism* means not round; *a* for "not," *stigmata* for "round." The surface of a "normal" eye is uniformly round, even if it is hyperopic or myopic. It has two directions, each called an axis; the axes usually are perpendicular, with one a horizontal axis and the other vertical. An astigmatic eye is not uniformly round; it is too steeply curved on one axis and too flat on the other.

Many people describe the astigmatic cornea as oval or football-shaped. Dr. Phillips demonstrates what astigmatism is like by squeezing the top and bottom of a tennis ball with the palms of his hands. As the patient sees it, the ball is now flattened "cross-ways" and more curved "up and down." This is how an astigmatic cornea appears. Consequently, light does not converge at a single point—whether short of, behind, or on the retina—but at two sep-

An eye with a cornea that is not round like a baseball, but instead oval like a football, is said to be astigmatic. People with astigmatism have difficulty with near and distance vision. Astigmatism is expressed as a minus or a plus number, depending on how the doctor was trained.

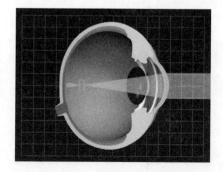

arate focal points. People with astigmatism experience blurred, shadowy, or doubled vision, both near and far.

Measured by strength or weakness of focusing power, astigmatism can be plus (+) or minus (−), depending on how the doctor was trained. In reality, it doesn't make any difference. The person making the glasses (or entering the information into the laser computer) just needs to pay attention to which way the prescription is written. The axis is written as 45 degrees, 90 degrees, 180 degrees, and so forth.

Of those people with astigmatism, most have regular astigmatism, meaning their corneas are not round but still have a regular known shape, like a football. Some people have an irregular astigmatism. A cornea with an irregular astigmatism has peaks and valleys at various points on the surface. Irregular astigmatism is more difficult to correct, although patients have the greatest success with semi-rigid, gas-permeable lenses, as these mask the irregular shape with a perfect piece of round plastic. There also are people whose corneas are symmetrically round but whose crystalline lenses are not, which results in a condition called lenticular astigmatism. Corrective lenses are prescribed to adjust for the total astigmatism present on both the cornea and the crystalline lens.

At this point, you have almost enough information to read your own lens prescription, but not quite. We haven't discussed how focusing power is measured.

Focusing Power

When we talk about vision and vision problems, we mean focus and focusing power. Focus refers to the convergence of light rays at a single point. In the eye, that point is the retina and, specifically, the macula. Focusing power is the ability of a medium to direct light rays to the point of focus, which is also expressed as the medium's light-gathering power, or "speed." When focusing a camera, the photographer determines the f-stop: the speed at which light will be gathered by the lens to achieve proper focus.

Anything through which light can pass has focusing power—water, plastic, and glass, for example. In the eye, light passes through the cornea. The shape of the cornea determines, in part, the point of focus. The cornea can be shaped with a knife, as in radial keratotomy, or with an excimer laser. By changing its shape, the surgeon changes the cornea's focusing power. As you read earlier, the crystalline lens also plays a role in focusing light, as does the tear film. If the medium through which light passes can be shaped, then the point of focus can be changed. That's why eyeglasses and contact lenses can be used to correct your vision. Lenses relatively thicker in the center than on the edges add power and magnification. Lenses relatively thinner in the center and thicker at the edges decrease power and magnification.

> *The cornea can be shaped, with a knife as in radial keratotomy, or with an excimer laser. By changing its shape, the surgeon changes the cornea's focusing power.*

Maybe you've noticed a temporary change in your vision after swimming under water or when you had tears or raindrops in your eyes or on your lenses. The water very briefly changed the focusing power of your cornea by bending the light differently as it entered your eye. Contact lenses work in this manner.

Diopters and Your Prescription

People with less than perfect vision are said to have refractive errors. They are measured in units called diopters, which refer to the amount of focusing power required to close the distance between the retina and the point at which light naturally focuses in your eye: the focal length.

Focal length is measured in ordinary units such as inches, feet, and meters, and in diopters, which are equal to the reciprocal (reverse) of the focal distance measured in meters. One diopter is equal to about one meter (3.28 feet or 40 inches); two diopters equal one-half of a meter (1.64 feet or 20 inches); three diopters equal one-third of a meter; and so on.

The greater your refractive error, the more focusing power you need. Two diopters of myopia require twice as much focusing assistance as one diopter for light to fall properly on the retina. Five diopters require five times as much focusing assistance.

If light naturally focuses precisely on the retina, then you have no refractive error, which is expressed as 0.00, and the cornea is said to be plano. An eye with no refractive error is said to be emmetropic. If light falls short of the retina, the measurement would be expressed as a minus number because the eye has too much focusing power (myopia), and corrective lenses have to reduce the focal power of the cornea. If the focal point were behind the retina, the measurement would be expressed as a plus number because corrective lenses are needed to add power (hyperopia).

So, a person with −4.00 diopters of myopia has better distance vision than a person with −6.00 diopters of myopia, but not as good as someone with −2.00 diopters of myopia. Similarly, a person with +4.00 diopters of hyperopia has near vision that is better than a person with +6.00 diopters of hyperopia, but not as good as someone with +2.00 diopters of hyperopia. Astigmatism also is measured in diopters. In prescriptions for corrective lenses diopters are measured in one-quarter (0.25) increments.

Your visual acuity is not your prescription, but there is a correlation. The following chart shows roughly how focusing power (refraction) relates to crispness of vision (visual acuity.)

	Refraction	Acuity
No or minimal refractive error	0.00 −0.50	20/20+ 20/30
Low myopia	−1.00 −2.00 −3.00 −4.00	20/50 20/150 20/250 20/400
Moderate myopia	−5.00 −6.00 −7.00	20/500 20/650 20/800
Extreme myopia	−8.00 −9.00	20/1000 20/1300

This should only be considered a rough guide to the correlation between your prescription and your uncorrected visual acuity. One-quarter of the U.S. population wears corrective lenses for distance vision. Some 80 percent of these people have a refractive error of −6.00 diopters or less. Only 2 percent of the lens-wearing population have refractive errors of greater than −9.00 diopters. But, of course, these people are the most handicapped by their condition. For them, myopia is more than a refractive error; it is a disease state and often can lead to other ocular health problems.

Reading Your Prescription

Now you are ready to look at the prescription your doctor gave you for corrective lenses and really understand what the numbers mean. Let's take a look at my prescription prior to having PRK five years ago.

	Sphere	Cylindrical	
O.D. (ocular dexter, or right eye)	−1.75	+1.50	88
O.S. (ocular sinister, or left eye)	−1.75	+1.00	88

The degree to which you are myopic or hyperopic appears in the first column under "Sphere" for spherical refractive error. I had −1.75 diopters of myopia in both my right (O.D.) and my left (O.S.) eye. How astigmatic you are is represented under the "Cylindrical" column for cylindrical refractive error. In my case, both my eyes had slight astigmatism. The 88 refers to the degree or the axis of the astigmatism. Think of it as the direction in which the football is turned. "Axis 90" refers to a vertical orientation. "Axis 180" refers to a horizontal orientation.

I elected to have monovision and left my left (nondominant) eye untreated. Currently, I have .50 diopter of myopia in my right eye with no astigmatism, and my left eye is unchanged from the prescription you just read. (See chapter 5 for a discussion of monovision.) However, now that I am growing increasingly presbyopic, I likely will have the astigmatism treated in my left eye to get rid of the shadows and sharpen my vision, still saving my eyesight for up close.

If you are over 40 and presbyopic, you might choose to wear bifocals. The amount of additional focusing power you need to read comfortably is written as an addition (add) to your prescription. Prescription pads vary, but it might have the word "Add" underneath the word "Distance," and in the "Sphere" column would appear numbers such as +1.50 or −2.00.

Best Spectacle-Corrected Visual Acuity

Now that you know what visual acuity means and how to read your prescription, here's another term you will hear if you decide to have laser vision correction: best spectacle-corrected visual acuity (BSCVA). This also is sometimes seen as BCVA, which means the same thing but the spectacle is dropped, maybe because it really doesn't matter whether the vision is corrected with glasses or contacts.

In any case, BSCVA refers to the best visual acuity a person can achieve with corrective lenses. If your uncorrected visual acuity is 20/400, but with glasses or contacts you can see as well as a normal person, then your BSCVA is 20/20. Many people, for any number of reasons, cannot be corrected to 20/20 even with lenses. Their BSCVA might be 20/25 or 20/30 and sometimes higher. But many other people can have their vision corrected with lenses, particularly with contact lenses, to better than 20/20. They might have visual acuity of 20/15 or even 20/10 when wearing their corrective lenses.

When evaluating patients for laser vision correction, doctors always measure their uncorrected visual acuity and their best corrected visual acuity to ensure that the proper refractive numbers are programmed into the laser's computer. This also helps the doctor to better evaluate the results following the treatment, as compared to the patient's best corrected vision before laser treatment.

A Simpler Way to Know

Of course, the simplest way to know if you are myopic or hyperopic is to look at your eyeglass lenses and at yourself in the mirror with your eyeglasses on. If the lenses of your glasses are thicker at the edges and thinner toward the center, you are myopic. If when you look at yourself in the mirror with your glasses on, your eyes appear small, or "beady," you are myopic.

If, on the other hand, your eyeglasses are thicker in the middle and thinner as the lenses spread out toward the frame, you are hyperopic. If when you look at yourself in the mirror with your glasses on, your eyes appear magnified, you are a hyperope.

Astigmatism isn't quite as easy to detect and may not be detectable at all just by looking at your lenses. However, if you hold your eyeglasses a little bit in front of you and rotate them like a steering wheel, you may be able to see images come into focus, become distorted, and come back into focus, depending on which part of the lens you look through.

Vision That's Good Enough

If the majority of people have some degree of refractive error, it begs the question: How come we don't see more people wearing eyeglasses? Well, besides the obvious answer that many people wear contact lenses, there also are many people walking around whose vision is less than perfect, but they don't necessarily wear eyeglasses or contact lenses, or they wear them only some of the time because their vision is "good enough."

Who determines whether vision is good enough? You do! My son Tim has −2.50 diopters of myopia in both eyes, with no astigmatism. He wears glasses to drive, watch television or movies, and to read the blackboard in school. Yet he is very comfortable walking around without his glasses much of the time. His brother, Sam, on the other hand, with −2.00 diopters of myopia in both eyes and slight astigmatism, wears his glasses most of the time. For Tim, good enough is slightly blurry. For Sam, good enough is crisp, sharp focus. For my husband who had −5.50 diopters of myopia in both eyes before his recent surgery, "good enough" was determined by circumstances. Around the house he was comfortable going without his glasses, although he couldn't see much, but leaving the house without them would have been disastrous.

People with moderate to high degrees of myopia or hyperopia and/or large amounts of astigmatism are usually completely dependent on their corrective lenses. For this group, poor vision is a safety-compromising handicap and "good enough" might mean simply reducing that total dependence. Even people with only slight refractive errors can become dependent on corrective lenses to function effectively and safely behind the wheel of an automobile, on the job, or when engaged in recreational activities.

For some people, good enough means accepting the necessity of wearing reading glasses in exchange for excellent distance vision. Others prefer to give up some clarity of distance vision to be able to read without glasses. The only person who can decide what's good enough regarding your vision is you. That's why the decision to have laser vision correction is such a personal decision. No one else can define for you what your optimum visual acuity is, given your lifestyle, profession, or personal preference.

Deciding If You're a Good Candidate

The very first thing that must be determined before you decide if you are a good candidate for laser vision correction is whether you have a refractive error (chances are you do if you are reading this book, but you never know). Then you will want to know exactly how much of a refractive error you have. And also of critical importance is knowing whether or not you have certain vision and general health conditions that would rule out refractive surgery. These are called contraindications.

The only way to determine whether you are a good candidate clinically is to visit your eye doctor for a thorough eye exam. (See chapter 5 for a review of what constitutes a comprehensive, preoperative eye examination.) If you don't have an eye doctor, have moved to a new area, or would prefer to visit someone new, you can locate an eye doctor who specializes in refractive surgery through any of the laser vision correction management companies such as TLC, LCA Vision, and Clear Vision. You should ask your friends, colleagues, or family members who have had laser vision correction who performed their surgery and whether they are satisfied with the results.

> *The only way to determine whether you are a good candidate clinically is to visit your eye doctor for a thorough eye exam.*

You also can "surf the Net." You might try visiting the Web sites of laser manufacturers such as VISX, Summit Technology, Bausch & Lomb Surgical, or LaserSight. Most of them have lists of doctors who perform refractive surgery. However, you should understand that the doctors listed on many of these Web pages are just doctors who have taken a laser-training course. The lists do not differentiate between a doctor who has done two LASIK procedures and one who has done 2,000. Ask your eye doctor to name two or three doctors whom he would let operate on his eyes, and then visit each of their offices and determine where you feel most comfortable.

You can do a Web search by typing in *refractive surgery, LASIK, PRK,* or *laser vision correction,* but be prepared for a mind-boggling list of sites. And always bear in mind that anyone can post anything on the Internet. So viewer, beware. Laser manufacturers' sites and those of physicians must adhere to strict regulatory guidelines for advertising and promotion of medical products; they are more likely to contain information that is accurate and verifiable.

Contraindications:
When Considering Refractive Surgery

There are some general guidelines to follow in determining whether you are a good candidate for laser vision correction and certain health conditions that are reason to take extra care in the decision-making process. For example, women who are pregnant or nursing should not have refractive surgery. They should wait at least six months after giving birth or weaning is completed. During pregnancy vision can fluctuate, and it takes several months after a woman has stopped nursing her child for vision to return to prepregnancy levels. Also, the medications taken in the form of eyedrops can potentially cause harm to the developing baby.

People with uncontrolled diabetes or diabetes-related vision problems need to check with their internist and their eye doctor before considering laser vision correction—as should people who suffer from autoimmune diseases, an uncontrolled vascular disorder, or a connective tissue disease.

Certain ocular health conditions must be ruled out before a person can have laser vision correction; these include glaucoma, retinal tears, and previous ocular surgery. People with pupils that are too large or corneas that are too thin also are not good candidates. These are ocular contraindications that will show up in a comprehensive preoperative eye examination. (See chapter 5 for a complete discussion of medical and ocular contraindications.)

Other than that, you must be 18 years of age or older and have had a stable prescription for at least one year; two years is better if you are closer to 18 than to 25. A stable prescription is one that has not changed by more than 0.50 diopters during the previous twelve-month period. So, if you are eager to reduce your dependence on, but not necessarily eliminate your need for, glasses or contact lenses, you might be an excellent candidate.

As you begin the decision-making process, you might want to consider the following questions from the LASIK Institute's Web site.

Do you have a strong desire to reduce your dependence on glasses?

Do your glasses or lenses interfere with your job, sports, or daily activities?

Do you clearly understand and accept the risks of surgery?

Do you clearly understand that the effects of LASIK are permanent and do not wear off?

Do you understand that refractive procedures require follow-up examinations at very specific intervals?

Do you have time to attend these examinations?

Are your expectations of refractive surgery realistic?

If you honestly answered yes to all of these questions and you know you are without any medical contraindications to refractive surgery, read on. Next you will learn how to find a laser vision correction team that will work with you to help you achieve the best possible visual results.

4

How Can I Find the Best Doctor?

"In real estate it's location, location, location," comments Bernie Haffey, vice president of marketing with Summit Technology, Inc. "In laser vision correction, and particularly when looking for a surgeon to perform LASIK, it's experience, experience, experience."

When asked about the most important thing that experience teaches a surgeon, Dr. Machat says emphatically: "Experience teaches a surgeon, first, how to avoid complications, and, second, how to manage complications in the rare instance when they do occur.

"You only have one pair of eyes," Dr. Machat cautions. "Do you want to have them surgically altered by someone who has done a dozen cases or someone who has performed thousands?"

In my work with TLC, I had the opportunity to watch experienced surgeons, as well as those just learning refractive surgery techniques. I also watched dozens of surgeons as they first held the microkeratome in their hands while sitting at the laser and treating animal eyes through the laser's microscope. I watched doctors as they treated their first human patients, and I can tell you that all of the surgeons held their breath as they made the first pass with the microkeratome. Every single surgeon had beads of sweat on his or her brow. Dr. Brint, who has trained hundreds of surgeons in refractive techniques, confirms my observation.

Many of these surgeon "trainees" had performed corneal transplants and/or cataract surgery for years prior to learning refractive surgery techniques. These were not newly minted doctors fresh from residency. In fact, one surgeon with ten years' experience performing cataract surgery walked away from his very first LASIK case, saying, "No more. From now on, I will refer all my refractive patients to someone who does this all the time. I don't have the nerves for this."

What I learned while facilitating surgeon training and by watching inexperienced and experienced surgeons is that this is not an easy procedure. Experienced surgeons make it look easy, and for them there is the ease that comes with repetition, but the learning curve for refractive surgery, and LASIK specifically, is a steep one.

> *Experienced surgeons make it look easy, and for them there is the ease that comes with repetition, but the learning curve for refractive surgery, and LASIK specifically, is a steep one.*

With each successful treatment, a surgeon gains confidence in his or her abilities and there is a subtle but dramatic change in behavior. The more patients surgeons treat, the more efficient in their movements they become. What separates the highly experienced from those with little experience is precision and confidence. Experienced surgeons waste no time in the execution of treatment. It is not because they are eager to move on to the next patient and earn a few more dollars, although some have been accused of this; it is because the more quickly they accomplish the correction, the better the outcome.

Explains Dr. Brint, "The cornea is 75 percent water. During surgery it begins to dry out almost immediately. The goal is to keep the eye in as close to its natural physiological state as possible because that is the condition under which treatment decisions were made, and because keeping the eye in its natural state results in less trauma to the eye."

Dr. Anthony Kameen adds, "It has been proven that the least amount of time spent in performing the treatment, the better the outcome."

Experienced surgeons have an efficiency of movement in the laser suite that could be described as ballet-like. My friends in Dr. Whitten's office compare it to conducting a symphony orchestra. Every step in the process is accomplished with exactness, with a precision of movement that is extraordinary to watch, in that it gives an appearance of effortlessness belying the complexity of the procedure. That appearance of effortlessness only comes with experience gained over time and through the completion of hundreds of successful procedures.

Contributing to that appearance of effortlessness is the support team that works with the surgeon in the laser room before a patient even enters the operating room. Each member of the team has a specific task to perform and each knows exactly what to do, how to do it, and when. But this only happens after the surgeon and his or her team has worked together on thousands of cases.

Patient Co-Management

Surgeons achieve that level of precision when they work with an equally experienced team that consists of primary eye-care doctors, patient consultants, ophthalmic technicians, laser technicians, and the entire administrative staff of the facility where surgery is performed. Every member of the team plays a critical role in achieving the best possible outcome for each patient. When you are ready to select a surgeon and a facility, a question you might ask is, "Does the doctor routinely work with the same staff or does the support staff change from day to day?"

Before I describe each member of the laser vision correction team, it is important to introduce a term you almost certainly have come across during the course of your research into laser vision correction. That term is *co-management*. It means, simply, that the ophthalmologist who performs surgery works closely with a primary eye-care doctor, usually an optometrist, but sometimes with a general ophthalmologist, in planning, treating, and following up with patients.

Some refractive surgeons do provide total care, but not many. And I can't think of a single highly experienced surgeon who does so, except those who have full-time optometrists on staff. They don't because it's not practical. A confident surgeon will tell you that the optometrists with whom they work are equally able to precisely determine a patient's refractive error. This is an optometrist's area of expertise. Optometrists specialize in vision problems and refractions. They fit glasses and contacts day in and day out, and increasingly they manage refractive surgery patients pre- and postoperatively. Ophthalmologists, on the other hand, specialize in diagnosing diseases of the eye and/or in the surgical correction of vision problems. They rarely do their own refractions.

Most busy surgeons co-manage patients with a number of different primary care doctors. They do so for the reason stated previously, but, most important, they co-manage because this is in the best interests of the patient. Optometrist David Sullins points out that "The doctor who has been caring for a prospective patient's vision over many, many years is in a much better position to help that patient make a decision about laser vision correction than is someone who is seeing them for the first time."

Co-management requires a high level of trust between the surgeon and the referring doctor. The surgeon must trust that the doctor's preoperative examination has been thorough and that no medical reasons exist dictating that the patient should not have surgery. The surgeon also must have a high level of trust that the patient's refractive error has been properly measured, to ensure a good outcome, although this is normally checked at the laser center by a second doctor. The surgeon should have confidence that the referring doctor is fully able to identify and manage postsurgical abnormalities.

On the other hand, referring doctors place extraordinary trust in surgeons and must have confidence that the surgeons will achieve excellent results, treat their patients well, and return to their practice satisfied patients. A good place to start your search for the best surgeon is to ask your primary eye-care doctor which surgeon or surgeons he or she refers to. Also, ask how many cases have been performed by the doctor(s). You might ask to speak with some of the doctor's patients who already have had laser vision correction.

The Laser Vision Correction Team

Trust is critical to successful outcomes, and that trust must exist between all members of the laser vision team, which typically include the following.

Ophthalmologist. An ophthalmologist is a doctor who has completed four years of college, four years of medical school, one year as an intern practicing general medicine or surgery, and three to four years in a residency program specializing in the diagnosis and treatment of diseases of the eye and visual problems. Some ophthalmologists also complete one or more specialty programs, called fellowships.

Fellowships offer comprehensive training in the treatment of one aspect of eye care, such as the cornea, the retina, or ocular disease.

Although some ophthalmology residencies now include study of refractive surgery, that is a fairly recent phenomenon. Prior to the October 1995 approval of the excimer laser by the FDA, any ophthalmologist with an interest in refractive surgery received training as part of a continuing medical education (CME) course or informally from another refractive surgeon. After that date, surgeons interested in using the excimer laser in refractive surgery were required to complete a certification program designed and administered by VISX or Summit Technologies, the two manufacturers then approved by the FDA for use in PRK.

> *Board certification is not a requirement for licensure, but a board-certified surgeon has evidence of subject mastery.*

Ophthalmologists are licensed by the state in which they practice and must pass an examination administered by a state board to receive a license. The State Board of Medical Examiners is responsible for monitoring medical care in the state and for identifying and disciplining doctors who are found to give substandard care. The American Board of Ophthalmology also certifies ophthalmologists who have completed a comprehensive examination on general ophthalmology. Board certification is not a requirement for licensure, but a board-certified surgeon has evidence of subject mastery. You might ask about board certification when making inquiries during your surgeon-selection process.

On its Web site, the American Board of Ophthalmology posts the following definition of an ophthalmologist:

Ophthalmologists are medical doctors specializing in the comprehensive care of the eyes and vision. They are the only practitioners medically trained to diagnose and treat all eye and visual problems, including vision services (glasses and contacts), and provide treatment and prevention of medical disorders of the eye, including surgical procedures.

Optometrist. Most people (70 percent, give or take) visit an optometrist for routine eye care, which includes obtaining prescriptions for corrective lenses. Optometrists typically attend four years of college and four years of optometry school, graduating with a doctor of optometry (O.D.). Optometrists also have the option, as do ophthalmologists, of completing fellowship programs in specific areas of treatment. Optometrists are licensed by the state in which they practice and must pass an exhaustive licensing examination. The American Optometric Association (AOA) defines optometrist as follows:

Doctors of optometry are independent primary health-care providers who examine, diagnose, treat, and manage diseases and disorders of the visual system, the eye, and associated structures, as well as diagnose related system conditions.

They examine the internal and external structure of the eyes to diagnose eye diseases like glaucoma, cataracts, and retinal disorders; systemic diseases like hypertension and diabetes; and vision conditions like nearsightedness, far-sightedness, astigmatism, and presbyopia. Optometrists also do testing to determine the patient's ability to focus and coordinate the eyes, and to judge depth and see colors accurately. They prescribe eyeglasses and contact lenses, low-vision aids, vision therapy, and medicines to treat eye diseases.

As an integral part of the laser vision correction team, optometrists provide a comprehensive preoperative examination to determine a patient's eligibility for the procedure and the degree of refractive error to be corrected. Optometrists refer patients to ophthalmologists for surgery. Only an ophthalmologist can perform refractive surgical procedures.

Adds Dr. Brint, "Optometrists who work closely with refractive surgeons have undergone many hours of rigorous training in postoperative care and in the recognition of early problems that may need to be referred back to the surgeon."

Ophthalmic Technicians. Good surgeons rely on the support of a highly skilled team of technicians to ensure a successful refractive outcome for every patient. These professionals are trained to operate all the ophthalmic equipment used in the course of a comprehensive preoperative eye exam, treatment, and postoperative care, including:

- Corneal topographer—also called a videokeratographer, the corneal topographer is used to take a picture of the surface of your eye and to generate a color map of the cornea showing where the cornea is steepest or deepest and how it is shaped. This procedure also rules out potential patients with vision problems such as keratoconus caused by uneven corneas.

- Pachymeter—a device used to measure the thickness of the cornea.

- Auto refractor—a machine that approximates your refractive error by "reading" your eye and prints out your prescription.

- Lensometer—a device that "reads" the prescription from the lenses of your eyeglasses.

- Phoropter—the monstrous-looking device mounted in front of an ophthalmic chair into which a patient peers while a doctor or technician asks, "Which is better, one or two?"

- Microkeratome—An instrument that is perhaps most critical of all, used to create the flap of tissue that is lifted during refractive surgery.

The use of each of the ophthalmic devices listed here is described in a discussion of the comprehensive preoperative examination in chapter 5.

The training and experience of ophthalmic technicians vary widely from facility to facility. Some ophthalmic technicians are certified by the Joint Commission on Allied Health Personnel in Ophthalmology (JCAPHO), although certification is not required to operate any of the previously named instruments. Others are members of the American Society of Ophthalmic Administrators (ASOA), a fellow organization of the American Society of Cataract and Refractive Surgeons (ASCRS), which provides continuing education and training for technicians who work with refractive surgeons.

Certified ophthalmic technicians (COT) have undergone a rigorous training regimen, including course work and "wet labs," which provides hands-on experience with instrumentation in a supervised setting.

Many ophthalmic technicians are trained by the surgeon with whom they work, and most take continuing education courses offered by professional associations with which they are affiliated. Device manufacturers provide technician training, and all of the laser companies provide training to ensure excellence of care.

Laser Technicians. The professionals who run the lasers at any provider facility are called laser technicians. Anyone who operates the laser is required to complete a training course designed and administered by the manufacturer of the laser he or she operates, or by the company's designee. In a large laser company such as TLC, the more experienced technicians train the new hirees. Laser technicians program the laser for desired correction, based on the refractive numbers provided to them by the surgeon.

Dr. Brint points out that "a surgeon arrives at the refractive numbers to be entered into the computer based on the patient's refractive error and age, as well as his or her experience with the laser being used. A number of factors must be considered, including altitude and humidity. Lasers in Denver, Colorado, which is at a high elevation and where the air is dry, behave differently than lasers in Miami, Florida, where it is humid and at sea level."

Laser technicians also monitor the laser's performance. They are responsible for checking the system at the beginning of each procedure day and between cases. One of the most important tasks required of them is to ensure that the laser is "firing" properly, that the beam is delivering energy consistently, and that it is properly aligned. In addition, the surgeon is able to immediately identify any inconsistency in energy delivery. Inconsistent energy delivery, called "hot spots," can result in more or less correction than intended. An improperly aligned beam can deliver energy to the wrong part of the cornea, also resulting in a less than desirable outcome.

Laser testing is a critical part of the technicians' training. Materials to conduct these tests are provided by the laser manufacturers, who also periodically sample test results to ensure continued proper functioning of the laser.

A question you might ask of a facility you are considering for treatment is: "How frequently do your technicians test the laser's performance?" If the answer is less than every patient, think about going somewhere else for treatment.

Patient Consultants. Although they are called by different titles at different facilities, the function they serve is the same. The patient consultant can make the difference between a good experience and a decision not to have the procedure. Patient consultants often are the first people prospective patients talk to as they begin the decision-making process. The role of the patient consultant is to be educator, counselor, cheerleader, and salesperson.

Patient consultants can answer many of your questions about the procedure, but they cannot dispense medical advice. That is, they can't tell you whether you are or are not a perfect candidate for refractive surgery; only a doctor can do that. If, as you begin your inquiry, you encounter a patient consultant who seems a bit too eager to "get you under the laser" or who tells you that you are a great candidate before you've had a complete eye exam, you might want to ask them how they are compensated. In some facilities, patient consultants receive a "bonus" for every patient they persuade to have laser vision correction. "However," adds Dr. Brint "the vast majority of patient consultants are primarily concerned with the education of the patient, and with achieving the best possible outcome for each patient, which sometimes means the patient does not have surgery."

Patient consultants can tell you about payment plans that may be available through the doctor or the facility where the procedure will be performed. Most providers of laser vision correction do try to make the surgery as affordable as possible by arranging flexible programs with area banks or with one of several nationwide financial services chains. (For more information about payment options, see chapter 8.)

Teamwork Delivers Better Results

Teamwork is essential to achieving excellent results consistently. It is imperative that the surgeon trusts the co-managing doctor's preoperative examination and that the surgeon trusts the skills of the team with which he or she works in the laser suite. That trust, of course, comes after many hours of working together. When a surgeon chooses a facility at which to perform refractive surgery, he or she is also choosing a level of quality and training of the support team.

These days, refractive surgeons have many options available to them. There are freestanding facilities that specialize in nothing but laser vision correction, some of which are owned and operated by management companies, others by hospitals, and some by investors that finance the laser purchase for a surgeon or group of surgeons. Some independent doctors and some group ophthalmology practices own or lease a laser that is shared by doctors within that group and that is sometimes made available to other surgeons on a pay-for-use basis.

Doctors who treat at a freestanding center might pay a fee to use the laser, which is owned by the company that manages the center. This is called an open-access facility. Open-access facilities usually provide a technician to operate the laser and might have ophthalmic technicians on staff to provide support as needed but, by and large, expect surgeons to bring with them any support staff they need.

Surgeons who own their own lasers, or jointly own one with a group of surgeons, hire and train their own surgical support staff. In those situations it is desirable that the staff be completely dedicated to laser vision correction.

Many doctors sign a contract with a management company that owns and operates the laser facility. The surgeon agrees to pay a facility fee, which is higher than that paid to an open-access facility because the management company provides administrative services as well. These centers often collect a "global fee" from the patient, subtract from that fee the amount the surgeon owes for use of the facility, and forward the remainder of the fee to the surgeon. (See chapter 8.) Management company–owned centers generally are fully staffed with optometrists, patient consultants, and ophthalmic and laser technicians. Generally speaking, surgeons sign up for a block of time during which they treat patients who have come through their practice and patients referred to them by other doctors.

Surgeons who treat with lasers owned by hospitals often rely on hospital personnel for surgical support. Surgeons who own their own lasers, or jointly own one with a group of surgeons, hire and train their own surgical support staff. In those situations it is desirable that the staff be completely dedicated to laser vision correction.

Some surgeons have dedicated their entire practice to refractive surgery; others offer laser vision correction as one of a menu of ophthalmic services. One isn't necessarily better than the other, but, it is often the case that specialists do one thing and do it extremely well. What's most important to know is how well trained the members of the team are and how well they work together in the delivery of patient care. Teams that work together frequently are much more likely to provide excellent care consistently than are those that come together only infrequently. You might want to ask the doctors you interview whether they work with more or less the same staff each time or if their support team changes from time to time.

The only way to find out where a particular surgeon will perform your surgery, and how frequently he or she works with the staff at that facility, is to ask. And while you are asking, the LASIK Institute, a nonprofit patient education organization funded by, but managed independently of, Summit Technology and the New England Eye Center, suggests that you also ask the following:

- Is this strictly a refractive surgery center or a full-service ophthalmic practice offering refractive surgery as one of its specialties?
- Will I have an opportunity to speak with the surgeon prior to surgery?

- Who will be my main contact at the office? (Surgeon? Nurse? Refractive Coordinator?)
- Who performs the follow-up examinations?
- What are the qualifications of the person providing follow-up care?

Training

We suggest you also ask what kind of training has been provided to the refractive support team, including the patient coordinator or consultant and the technicians.

Other than the surgeon, no member of a refractive surgery team is required to obtain any specific certification or license. As mentioned previously, to be called a certified ophthalmic technician, a person must pass a certification exam administered by JCAPHO; however, no company that we know of requires technicians to be certified to become part of a laser vision correction surgical support team.

Bausch & Lomb Surgical, distributors of the most commonly used microkeratome, recommends that the person who supports the surgeon in the laser room attend the same users' course that the surgeon is required to attend. But attendance is not mandatory for the assistant. Although there are many laser vision correction continuing education (CE) courses available to optometrists, attendance at such a course is not required to provide pre- and post-operative patient care to laser vision correction patients.

Explains David Sullins, O.D., "Most optometrists who are contemporarily trained probably have the skills and instrumentation needed to do what is necessary, but patients should ask their doctor about continuing education. Someone interested in laser vision correction should make sure that the doctor who is doing his or her pre-op work-up and post-op care has made a commitment to life-long learning. Patients have a right to know whether or not doctors have read the current literature or that they have attended courses that will help them recognize atypical healing patterns, for example. Further training isn't required, but any doctor who wants to sleep at night needs to make that commitment to him- or herself and to the patient."

Most optometrists do attend one or more continuing education (CE) programs prior to referring patients for refractive surgery. For example, optometrists affiliated with TLC Laser Eye Centers are invited and encouraged to attend its National Surgeons Training Course, which is offered three times a year at different locations around the country. TLC also provides training for optometrists at each of its centers throughout North America. Having an affiliation with a company that offers continuing education can be of enormous benefit to optometrists and ophthalmologists alike.

Another opportunity available to optometrists is VISX University, a two-day CE program developed by VISX Inc. to familiarize optometrists with all aspects of refractive surgery and patient management. Many private-practice doctors gain several hours of ongoing refractive education on a quarterly basis.

Required Training

In fact, only surgeons are required to complete a specific training program prior to using the excimer laser. When the FDA approved the excimer laser for use in PRK, it mandated that surgeons intending to use the excimer laser in refractive surgery attend a manufacturer-sponsored certification course.

Consequently, VISX and Summit Technology have in their employ training coordinators who travel anywhere a laser is installed for the purpose of training technicians to operate the laser and surgeons to operate and program the laser and master the steps required to complete a PRK procedure.

Technicians spend four to six hours learning the fundamentals of excimer laser technology, how the laser works, safety precautions, emergency response procedures, and routine maintenance chores to ensure that the laser continues to operate properly.

The surgical training programs consist of a slide presentation that includes the fundamentals of laser technology, the effect of the laser beam on tissue, a review of surgical technique, common side effects, possible complications, and expected outcome. A video of live procedures is part of the program, as is a hands-on "wet lab," during which trainees perform PRK on animal or cadaver eyes. Surgeons who are certified by the laser manufacturer teach these courses.

> *Surgeons are not required by the FDA or any other regulatory body to be trained in the use of the microkeratome to perform LASIK.*

Certification is granted only after a surgeon has performed at least one PRK procedure on a human patient under the supervision of an experienced laser surgeon, called a proctor. That is the extent of required training.

Surgeons are not required by the FDA or any other regulatory body to be trained in the use of the microkeratome to perform LASIK. However, microkeratome manufacturers are keenly aware that use of the product by a surgeon requires great skill and exposes the company to product liability claims. Consequently, manufacturers require surgeons to attend training courses and sometimes will not sell them the device or other equipment until training is complete.

Most surgeons who perform LASIK have attended at minimum a two-day program, which consists of six hours of lecture and four to six hours in a "wet lab," in which they practice on animal or cadaver eyes that have been rejected for possible corneal transplants. In the first part of the wet lab the doctor uses the microkeratome while sitting at a table operating on a "dummy" head. Later, the doctor actually treats pigs' eyes bought from a slaughterhouse, under the laser. During the wet lab the doctor also learns how to put together and take apart the microkeratome, how to ensure the device is operating smoothly, how to check for any defects, and how to clean all moving parts. Most important, doctors observe experienced surgeons. Proctored procedures are not required but are advised.

Informal Training

Few doctors would consider themselves refractive-surgery ready with so little practice and so little supervision. Most avail themselves of the innumerable continuing medical education courses offered at such professional association meetings as the American Academy of Ophthalmology (AAO), the American Society of Cataract and Refractive Surgeons (ASCRS), and the International Society of Refractive Surgeons (ISRS). And virtually all refractive surgeons have at one time or another sought out a more experienced surgeon with whom they compare nomograms, discuss a specific technique, and learn how to avoid and manage complications.

Surgeons who are affiliated with laser center companies have an advantage over those in solo practice, in that most laser center companies offer continuing education and training as part of their doctor-support services. In addition, the surgeons often participate in conference calls and meetings in which technology, technique, and outcomes are discussed.

For example, shortly after LASIK came into more wide-spread use, doctors affiliated with TLC began noticing an unusual complication in a very few patients. The corneas of these patients became cloudy and, when viewed under magnification, had the appearance of swirling sand. This problem has come to be known as Sands of the Sahara. Within days, every surgeon treating at a TLC center, and every referring doctor, was told about this complication and how to treat it. (See chapter 7 for a more complete discussion of complications.) Doctors treating independently might not learn of this problem until they encountered it for themselves, read about it in a professional journal, or heard about it at an association meeting. The capacity for instantaneous communication can be a sight-saving benefit of affiliation with a larger organization.

Specialists

Most ophthalmologists are general practitioners, diagnosing and treating diseases of the eye and vision problems. Some specialize in such specific areas of treatment as retina, glaucoma, pediatrics, cataracts, or cornea, and now refractive surgery. No area of specialization necessarily is better preparation for a move into refractive surgery than any other, except perhaps those specialties that require surgical skills.

Some surgeons will make much of the fact that they are cornea-trained. What that means is that they have attended at least one fellowship program that focused exclusively on diseases that affect the eye, such as infections, allergic conditions, ocular surface problems, and hereditary disorders. Ophthalmology residencies provide training in corneal transplantation; corneal fellowships offer additional transplantation training and also cover normal and abnormal corneal healing responses. Until the last two or three years, most corneal fellowships did not cover refractive surgery and, therefore, surgeons had to take the same postgraduate CME courses as other ophthalmologists.

Being a corneal specialist doesn't necessarily make a doctor a better refractive surgeon; however, many of them also perform corneal transplants, for which the same fine motor skills are required, as is adeptness at performing delicate surgery under a microscope. Ophthalmic surgeons who routinely perform cataract surgery have developed the same fine motor skills and level of comfort with surgery performed under a microscope as do surgeons who perform corneal transplants. Many surgeons will try to persuade patients that prior experience in one specialty or another makes them more suited to perform refractive surgery. The only prior surgical experience that makes a significant difference in refractive surgery outcomes is prior refractive surgical experience.

Even a cursory investigation of the United States's most experienced refractive surgeons will quickly reveal that most have a long history of involvement with refractive surgery. Some were clinical investigators for one of the laser manufacturers on their own or in a teaching hospital; others built a significant refractive practice offering RK.

Virtually all of today's highly regarded refractive surgeons are "early adopters." Maybe it's a concept you are familiar with. In chapter 2, we discussed early adopters in terms of patients who sought treatment outside the United States prior to FDA approval of the excimer laser for use in PRK. Early adopters are people who embrace new ideas or new technology long before the vast majority of the population is even aware that it exists.

Refractive surgery's early adopters are, by and large, self-taught. Before the laser was approved for commercial sale in the United States, many of today's best-known refractive surgeons were the original clinical investigators for manufacturers submitting premarketing applications to the FDA. Many of these surgeons also traveled to South

America, Europe, or Canada to learn from surgeons in those countries. When the laser was approved, they were the first to treat patients in the United States.

Questions to Ask

As laser vision correction becomes more widely accepted and ever more widely available, competition for patients will increase. The airwaves and print media will be saturated with advertisements featuring smiling people, presumably satisfied patients.

The ads will try to persuade potential patients that this or that doctor is better able to perform refractive surgery for any number of reasons. Cornea specialists will tout their corneal training and cataract surgeons their surgical skill. Growing numbers of doctors have participated in or are currently participating in clinical trials for different laser manufacturers. They will use that experience as a point of differentiation between themselves and "Doctor X" around the corner or at another center. Participation in clinical trials doesn't necessarily mean the doctor is experienced or uniquely qualified to perform refractive surgery. (See chapter 10 for a discussion of the FDA approval process and clinical trials.)

> *The most important question a prospective patient can ask a surgeon is, How many PRK and LASIK procedures have you performed?*

Don't be fooled by the claim of superior skill based on participation in clinical trials. Some of the earliest refractive surgeons, the true pioneers, such as Stephen Brint, Dan Durrie, Stephen Slade, James Salz, Mark Speaker, Jeffery Machat, and Mark Whitten, can rightfully make such an assertion, but they are few and far between. And today it doesn't really matter. Many surgeons have gained the necessary skills to perform refractive surgery since the laser was approved.

When it comes right down to it, the only skill that matters is the doctor's skill with refractive surgery. The only way to know how good the doctor is to ask questions, lots of questions.

While conducting research for this book, I talked with hundreds of people, patients, doctors, representatives of laser manufacturers, facility administrators, and others in the industry. Whatever else I asked them about, I always wanted to know: What are the most important questions prospective patients can ask to determine if the doctor they are considering as their surgeon is qualified?

To a person, regardless of their interest in refractive surgery, they all said the same thing: The most important question a prospective patient can ask a surgeon is, How many PRK and LASIK procedures have you performed?

There are many other questions a prospective patient should ask, but how many LASIK procedures the surgeon has performed is the most important of them. Beyond that, prospective patients should ask doctors about outcome. Be specific in asking about LASIK and/or PRK because many surgeons will exaggerate the number of refractive procedures they have performed by including RK and cataract surgery.

You should ask questions like, What percentage of patients treated by you achieve visual acuity of 20/40 or better, 20/20 or better? And you should ask surgeons how they track their outcomes. Any surgeon who can readily produce charts and graphs probably is monitoring patient results, although numbers can be deceiving. Furthermore, doctors are not required to monitor patient outcomes, and there is no established national standard, so comparing one surgeon's data to another can potentially be misleading.

The best advice here is, If it seems too good to be true, it probably is.

Another good question is, What percentage of your patients experience a complication? As you may remember from earlier in the book, every doctor occasionally has a patient with a complication during surgery or recovery. If, when you ask about complications, the doctor or the doctor's staff tells you that the doctor has never had a complication, walk away. If they aren't telling the truth about that, you have to wonder what else they aren't being truthful about.

Dr. Machat had a patient ask: "What is the second-worst complication that could happen?" And says Dr. Machat, "When you think about it, that was very smart. The worst possible complication, going blind, is highly unlikely, but the second worst is a little more likely. Now you are talking on a whole different level and you can address with patients all those things that could happen that might compromise the quality of their vision but will not leave them blind."

Prospective patients should ask about the experience of the laser support team, about the type of laser used, and how often the laser is tested for performance. Dr. Jim Thimons suggests that patients find out about laser maintenance and treatment protocol by asking such questions as "Does the surgeon use a different microkeratome blade for each patient or is the same blade used over and over again? How often is the laser tested for beam performance? When is the last time the surgeon did a clinical audit of his or her results?"

In the back of this book you will find appendix D "Tough Questions to Ask the Doctor." It is adapted from questions posted on the Internet by an organization called the Council for Refractive Surgery Quality Assurance (CRSQA), a nonprofit, privately funded refractive surgery educational organization.

A Web site to visit is that of the LASIK Institute (www.lasikinstitute.com), a nonprofit educational organization funded by, but independent of, Summit Technology Inc. They, too, suggest questions to ask to determine whether the surgeon you are considering is the best doctor for you. Some of refractive surgery's earliest pioneers are members of the Institute's board of directors, including this book's co-author, Stephen Brint.

The Search Begins

Where do you start looking for an experienced surgeon? First, ask your primary eye-care doctor. He or she very likely refers to one or more refractive surgeons and is probably in the best position to know which doctor would be right for you. Ask friends, coworkers, or family members who have had the procedure or who know someone who has. Call a laser vision correction center in your area and ask to speak with a patient coordinator or patient consultant. "Surf the Net," but beware. Anyone can post anything; it doesn't have to be true. Visit the Web sites of the different professional associations mentioned earlier, such as the American Optometric Association, AAO, ASCRS, and ISRS.

Respond to advertisements or go to the Yellow Pages. Once you make that first call, bring this book along with you, earmarked to the section on questions to ask. Then ask those questions and more. The best doctors are proud of their skill, proud of their results, and happy to answer all of your questions.

A Refractive Surgeon Chooses a Refractive Surgeon

Stephen F. Brint

When I decided to have LASIK, I looked for the following:

1. An expert who had done thousands of cases.

2. A surgeon who teaches around the world and is well respected by peers.

3. Someone who has successfully handled lots of complications (mostly from other surgeons).

4. Someone who is meticulous regarding the whole experience and who:

   - Has expert microkeratome knowledge,
   - Understands all the nuances of the laser and how it behaves with changing humidity and other environmental concerns
   - Has a warm, friendly, professional staff.

5. The kind of laser was irrelevant. I trust the surgeon to use what he or she feels is best.

This is what I looked for and found in Steve Slade, my good friend as well as someone with whom I have worked, teaching other surgeons around the world.

5

What's the First Step?

Now that you have some guidelines on finding a good doctor, you're ready to take the next step in your laser vision correction journey: You're ready for the preoperative consultation and examination.

If you wear corrective lenses, you have had a comprehensive eye examination at some time in your life. You may even have one every year. People whose refractive errors are high (greater than −9.00 diopters of myopia or +6.00 diopters of hyperopia) often have an annual exam at their own initiative or on the recommendation of their eye doctors because they are at greater risk for other ocular (eye) health problems.

However, even though an annual eye exam, like regular dental checkups, is advisable, most of us don't visit an eye doctor unless we have a problem. In fact, many people who wear corrective lenses can't remember when they last visited an eye doctor or whether they visited an optometrist or an ophthalmologist. If you're in that group, expect to undergo a thorough evaluation that includes a complete medical history before the doctor makes any recommendation about laser vision correction.

If you are among those people who regularly visit an eye doctor and have had the same eye doctor for many years, the preoperative examination probably won't include a medical history, because the doctor already has that in your file. Based on when you had your last eye exam, the doctor may or may not complete all of the following tests prior to making his or her recommendation. This will depend on when he or she last checked for each of the ocular conditions that may or may not preclude refractive surgery as a vision correction alternative.

Making the Appointment

When scheduling an appointment for your preoperative examination, make sure you arrange it for a time when you can be relaxed and not feel pressured to get to your next appointment or to pick up the children. The exam itself takes time, but you also may find that the consultation raises questions. You want to ensure that you have plenty of time to listen to the answers to those questions and to formulate any new ones.

The decision to have laser vision correction is a big step. Before taking that step, you need to understand how your vision, and your life, might change. Talking to former patients can help you in your decision-making process, but

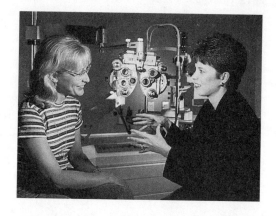

Doctor discusses laser vision correction with prospective patient. Ophthalmic equipment in the background is a phoropter, the device used to determine a patient's refractive error.

your experience won't be the same as those of your friends, coworkers, or family members. So it's important that you really listen and understand what the doctor and the doctor's staff tell you about the procedure, its benefits, and its potential complications.

> *The decision to have laser vision correction is a big step. Before taking that step, you need to understand how your vision, and your life, might change.*

Dr. Machat tells the following story to illustrate why it's important for each patient to pay full attention during the pre-op exam and consult. "I treated a close personal friend. His surgery was uneventful and his vision quickly settled in at 20/20. I then treated his wife, two of his brothers, and a sister. All did equally well. Then I treated his brother-in-law and had a complication, and the procedure had to be aborted. The man was devastated. He was depressed because even though I had explained to him that these things do happen, he was convinced it would not happen to him because nothing had happened to any of his relatives. What made it even worse was while he was healing, and waiting to attempt the procedure again, I treated another relative who also came through with no trouble and excellent results. I tell this story to illustrate how important it is that every single person be involved with his or her own treatment and not expect things to be the way they were for anyone else."

During the preoperative exam and consultation, the doctor will describe in some detail the benefits of laser vision correction and, even more important, the risks. He or she will discuss what to expect during the procedure and during your recovery; the common side effects; and the less common, but still possible, complications. It's a lot to take in. You will want to make time to really listen to the doctor so that you can make an informed choice about refractive surgery. Dr. Kameen recommends that a prospective patient bring a spouse, partner, or friend with them to the preoperative examination to help them process and understand the information.

In fact, it's a good idea when making that first appointment to tell the receptionist at the doctor's office or laser center that you are calling to make an appointment for a preoperative examination to determine your eligibility for laser vision correction. That way, the staff can give you any special instructions, such as to bring a pair of sunglasses because your eyes will be dilated and you will be very sensitive to light for an hour or so afterward.

Also, if you are certain that you want to have the procedure and this examination is for the purpose of ensuring candidacy, then the doctor likely will want you to stop wearing your contact lenses well ahead of the scheduled appointment. If the receptionist doesn't mention removing your contact lenses, ask if this is necessary.

Most doctors and laser vision correction centers recommend that prospective patients who regularly wear soft contact lenses stop wearing lenses and switch to eyeglasses at least one week prior to the initial examination. Wearers of hard or gas-permeable lenses generally are asked to stop wearing lenses for at least three weeks to a month prior to the initial examination. Some doctors suggest first a switch to soft lenses and later to eyeglasses, but that's a matter of personal preference for the patient. The important thing is that the eye be allowed to return to its natural shape before any treatment decisions are made.

This is very important. Contact lenses, even soft lenses, change your corneal reading, however temporarily. That change will affect the outcome of your eye examination. Performing surgery based on an eye examination conducted just after a patient has removed his or her contact lenses could very well result in an overcorrection. (See chapter 7 for a discussion of risks and complications.)

It can take weeks and possibly months for a person's eye to return to its natural shape after wearing hard contact lenses for a long period of time. So, as unhappy as you might be wearing eyeglasses for a few weeks, think of how much unhappier you will be if your postsurgery vision is affected by your failure to remove your contact lenses in good time.

By telling the receptionist or laser vision coordinator about your plans to have laser vision correction, you enable the staff to prepare in advance for your arrival. Also, many doctors send prospective laser vision correction patients a packet of educational material to read prior to the appointment. Dr. Kennedy notes that "The information obtained prior to your preoperative exam is extremely valuable in helping you prepare a list of questions. For one thing it might help reduce the amount of time you spend in the doctor's office, and for another it is always better to discuss any concerns you have before surgery, rather than afterward."

General Health

When you arrive for your appointment, you can expect to fill out the paperwork that is usually required when visiting a doctor for the first time. Also, before anyone even looks at your eyes, a member of the doctor's staff will ask you for a complete medical history. There are some diseases, just as there are some ocular conditions, that rule out laser vision correction. As mentioned in the previous chapter, these are called contraindications.

As optometrist Cynthia Wike explains: "Generally, when we screen a candidate for laser vision correction, there is a full range of tests that we do to ensure that the individual is a good candidate for the procedure. We look for signs of ocular disease such as cataracts, glaucoma, and retinal tears and for debilitating systemic diseases that compromise a person's healing response or could potentially affect his or her vision. Basically, healthy patients with healthy eyes make the best candidates."

Among the health conditions that might rule out refractive surgery are diabetes, collagen vascular diseases, and autoimmune or immunodeficiency diseases such as lupus, rheumatoid arthritis, AIDS, and scleroderma. Each of these diseases affects a person's healing response and, in some cases, can cause serious vision problems. But don't conclude on your own that you are not a candidate for refractive surgery. For example, many people whose diabetes is under control have had their vision successfully corrected with the laser. And as Dr. Kennedy reminds patients, "Only the surgeon can tell you for sure if you are or are not a candidate, perhaps after conferring with your personal physician about your health condition."

A good rule of thumb for an eye examination, as with any health exam, is to tell the doctor about any medications you are taking, including commonly prescribed drugs.

As mentioned in chapter 3, women who are pregnant or are nursing should wait until at least six months after giving birth or weaning the baby before having refractive surgery. Pregnancy often causes a change in vision. Elevated hormone levels also affect a woman's healing response. Therefore, any correction achieved during pregnancy will almost certainly require a second procedure when the body returns to its prepregnancy state.

When the excimer laser was first approved for use in PRK, keloid formation was included as a contraindication for refractive surgery. You are a keloid former if cuts and surgical incisions result in prominent large scars that do not go away. A history of keloid formation was believed to cause healing problems with PRK; however, many keloid formers have since had LASIK and have no higher incidence of healing problems than do non–keloid formers.

Some medications also affect vision and can cause postsurgical scarring or result in infiltrates (tiny little flecks) under the corneal flap. Among these are Accutane (generic name, isoretinoin), used to treat acne; Cordarone (generic name, amiodarone), prescribed for heart disease and for arthritis; and Imitrex (generic name, sumatriptan), prescribed for migraine headaches.

A good rule of thumb for an eye examination, as with any health exam, is to tell the doctor about any medications you are taking, including commonly prescribed drugs such as antihistamines or other allergy medications, birth control pills, and thyroid pills. Also tell the doctor about any medication to which you are allergic. Although you will be completely awake during your procedure, your eyes will be made numb with eyedrops. Just before and after surgery, you also will be given antibiotic and anti-inflammatory eyedrops, one to protect against infection and the other to minimize postsurgical swelling. You should be asked about allergies to medication, but if you're not asked, then you should volunteer the information. It's always better to be safe than sorry.

Ocular Health

A number of eye conditions may rule out refractive surgery. Again, these are general guidelines; the only way to know for sure whether you are a candidate is to have a thorough examination and to discuss with the doctor any health problems that you think might be cause for concern.

Among the ocular health conditions that may contraindicate refractive surgery are glaucoma, cataracts, herpes, diabetic retinopathy, keratoconus (steepening and thinning of the cornea), retinal tears, macular degeneration, and progressive myopia.

The size of the pupil can play a very critical role in the final outcome. Explains Dr. Kennedy: "The pupil is the black opening that allows light into the eye. The average pupil is about 5 mm to 6 mm, and the laser creates an opening (optical zone) of around 5 mm. If your pupil opening is greater than 6 mm and the optical zone created by the laser is 5 mm, it is possible that you will have problems with your vision after surgery, particularly at night." Consequently, too-large pupils might rule out refractive surgery, at least for now.

Lasers used most widely in the United States today are broad beam lasers, which means that the laser energy is delivered uniformly across the optical zone. In order to flatten the cornea to correct a myopic refractive error, more tissue has to be removed from the center of the optical zone than from the edges. Hyperopic corrections are accomplished by doing the opposite, by removing more tissue from the perimeter of the optical zone than from the center.

To achieve this, the laser's aperture, or opening, widens as the procedure progresses, ultimately delivering the required amount of laser energy to accomplish the desired correction. This results in very subtle gradations of correction. For people with very large pupils, the pupil may be larger than the treated zone, allowing uncorrected light to enter the pupil, causing vision problems such as glare and halos around bright lights. This phenomenon is particularly noticeable at night when the pupil is fully dilated and can make such activities as night driving more challenging. VISX Inc. and Summit Technology both manufacture broad beam lasers. Of course, the technology always is being perfected, and both companies are continuously improving laser energy beam delivery to create a smoother and larger corneal treatment surface.

Some lasers currently being tested will eliminate this problem by delivering the full amount of laser energy to the cornea in a random pattern with a "flying spot." These lasers' apertures are 1 to 2 mm wide, but they can be programmed to deliver energy to an optical zone of 10 mm. What's more, because the energy is delivered in a random circular pattern, the corneal surface in the treatment zone is smoother than a surface created by a broad beam laser. Because the gradations, or stair-step, problem has been eliminated, people with large pupils will have no greater likelihood of experiencing glare or halos than will any other refractive patient. In October, 1999, LaserSight Technologies received FDA approval for its "flying spot" laser. Since then, two other manufacturers of "flying spot" lasers, Autonomous Technologies and Bausch & Lomb Surgical, have received approval.

If you have any of these ocular conditions, it is very likely that you already know that you have them; however, many are asymptomatic, which means you can have the condition without experiencing any visual problems. Therefore, if the condition is not sufficiently advanced to result in vision loss, you may not know that you have the condition.

The pre-op exam is designed to discover these ocular health problems and to determine the degree of your refractive error, which is, of course, critical to a good outcome. When the FDA approved the excimer laser for use in PRK, the review panel recommended that patients be required to have a stable refraction for at least one year prior to having laser vision correction. A stable refraction means that the amount of your refractive error has not changed more than half a diopter (0.50 diopter) in a twelve-month period.

It's a good idea to bring a copy of your last prescription with you to your pre-op exam if you are seeing a doctor who has never examined you before. If you don't have it—and most of us don't; after all, who saves eyeglass or contact lens prescriptions?—you can obtain your prescription by calling the doctor who performed your last eye examination or the optician who filled the prescription. Certain doctors and some optical shops are reluctant to provide this information over the telephone and may even try to persuade you to come in for an exam to obtain a new reading. You don't have to. Information about the results of any health exam belong to the patient, not the doctor. They are required to provide you with that information.

The Pre-Op Exam

After a discussion of your general and ocular health, the doctor's staff will begin a series of tests. The order in which these tests are given is mostly a function of the availability of technicians and equipment, not a prescribed formula. However, you will have both a manifest refraction (without eyedrops) and a cycloplegic refraction (with eyedrops). The manifest refraction is performed first.

Refraction is the test given to measure your refractive error and to determine your uncorrected visual acuity (UCVA) and your best corrected visual acuity (BCVA)—that is, the very best you are able to see when wearing corrective lenses. It is that part of the exam when the doctor or technician has you peer into the phoropter and then flips lenses in front of your eyes, asking, "Which is better, one or two, two or three?" The manifest refraction is completed without dilating your pupils.

The second refraction is called a cycloplegic refraction and is accomplished using eyedrops, called cycloplegic agents, which ensure that your pupils remain fully dilated.

A cycloplegic refraction gives doctors a truer reading of your refractive error because it temporarily paralyzes the focusing muscle; thus, you are not able to adjust or accommodate to make things more clear. Usually, the results from a manifest refraction and cycloplegic refraction are pretty close, within half a diopter. But sometimes they're not. Then the doctor or technician may repeat both tests again at a later date.

If you wear corrective lenses, you are undoubtedly very familiar with both a manifest and a cycloplegic refraction because the doctor uses the results of these tests to write your eyeglass or contact lens prescription. You may or may not have had the other tests that will be described further on during your last regular eye exam. The equipment used in a preoperative exam includes:

Corneal topography, also called video keratography. A machine called a corneal topographer is used to create a computer-generated map of your cornea. The technician will ask you to sit on a stool in front of a very high

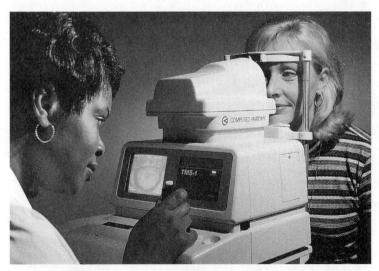

Prospective patient stares at the Placido target in the corneal topographer. The device will produce a computer-generated, four-color map of the cornea's surface.

tech–looking machine, place your chin on the curved metal rest, and stare into the series of black rings on a white background that grow increasingly smaller toward the center. This is called a Placido disk target, named for the person who first mapped the corneal surface in the 1880s. He or she will ask you to keep your eyes wide open and not to blink. Within seconds the machine will have taken a picture of the surface of your eye, plotting between 6,000 and 8,000 points on the cornea. The result is a four-color map of the cornea.

This map is used to determine the type of astigmatism you have, if any, and to learn where the cornea is steepest and flattest, aiding the surgeon in determining how to program the laser. The doctor also uses this map to discover whether a patient has keratoconus, which can rule out refractive surgery.

In addition, some doctors might take a measurement with a *keratometer*, which measures the curvature of the central 3 mm of the cornea. It is extremely precise but limited in its measurement. Corneal topographers cover a

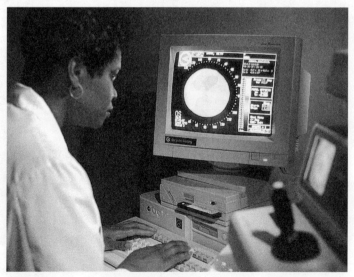

The technician prepares to print out the corneal map that appears on the screen of the corneal topographer.

much wider range. The two may be used to complement each other.

Slit Lamp. This is an ophthalmic instrument that you almost certainly are familiar with. Usually, the slit lamp is in the room—also called an examination lane—where the doctor performs his or her exam. It is a high-powered microscope that provides the doctor with a magnified view of the front of your eye. When the machine is in use, your chin is in the chin rest, and you are staring at a very bright light. The doctor may point to a spot to the side or just ahead and ask you to look in that direction.

Slit lamp exams are conducted primarily to check for cataracts, for evidence of glaucoma, and for scarring of the cornea (which would be evident on the map generated by the corneal topographer as well). The doctor also checks for such conditions as anterior basement membrane dystrophy and corneal vascularization—the presence of new blood vessels, which can be an indication of other problems. A special lens may allow the doctor to use the slit lamp to check the back of the eye, the retina, especially for fine details.

You may hear the doctor or technician talk about a *fundus* exam. This is an examination of the back of your eye. The doctor is checking for holes in the retina or signs of degeneration and for macular disease. These tests are usually conducted while your pupil is dilated.

A *tonometry* is taken to measure intraocular pressure to rule out glaucoma.

Corneal pachymeter. This device measures the thickness of your cornea. It is a critical component of a thorough preoperative exam. In refractive surgery, the doctor removes corneal tissue to achieve the desired correction, but there must be enough corneal tissue remaining to ensure continued ocular health and good vision. On average, the cornea is between 500 to 600 microns thick. Refractive surgery removes anywhere from 10 to 160 microns of tissue.

Obviously, the higher the refractive error, the more tissue is removed. People with high degrees of myopia or hyperopia also frequently need to have more than one procedure to reach the desired correction. This is called an enhancement, a retreatment, or is sometimes euphemistically referred to as a "tweaking" or "fine-tuning." Because every single person heals differently, it is not possible to say that people who fall in this or that range will or won't need to be retreated to achieve desired correction. But generally speaking, patients with low to moderate refractive errors are less likely to need an enhancement than are patients with higher refractive errors.

> *People with high degrees of myopia or hyperopia also frequently need to have more than one procedure to reach the desired correction.*

In the early days, before the lasers had been approved for use in hyperopia, surgeons tended to err on the extremely conservative side. When planning a desired correction, they would anticipate falling somewhat short of plano (no refractive error) to ensure that they did not overcorrect the patient, which would cause the once nearsighted patient to become farsighted. Retreatment rates were significantly higher for all surgeons. Now, farsightedness can be treated and surgeons are more comfortable targeting zero refractive error, because overcorrection is easily remedied.

Today, it is reasonable to expect lower enhancement rates than previously. Highly experienced surgeons have lower retreatment percentages, as they learn with each procedure how to adjust their nomograms, or treatment formulas, according to age, corneal curvature, humidity, and so forth. When interviewing doctors, ask about retreatment or enhancement rates; 10 to 20 percent is within the normal range.

If there is not sufficient corneal tissue remaining after the initial procedure, then a retreatment may not be possible. Doctors take this into consideration when making a recommendation about refractive surgery.

Other vision tests that will be performed during the pre-op exam include one to determine which eye is dominant. This is important if you decide to have surgery on only one eye at a time, in which case the surgeon probably will treat the nondominant eye first. If you elect to have monovision, you probably will have the dominant eye treated for distance vision and leave the other eye nearsighted for reading. (See "Treatment Decisions," later in this chapter.) To test for dominance, the technician or doctor might ask you to pretend to aim a gun or hold close to your eye a piece of paper with a small hole in it. The dominant eye is the eye you instinctively use first.

A *pupilometer* will be used to measure the size of your pupil when it is naturally dilated in a dark room. As mentioned earlier, people with unusually large pupils may have difficulty with glare and halos after refractive surgery. The doctor may check for *contrast sensitivity*, which is the ability of the eye to distinguish images of varying degrees of blackness. Loss of contrast sensitivity is a potential side effect of PRK and LASIK, so the doctor may set a baseline measurement, especially if you are involved in a study. It's also important for the doctor to determine how effectively your eyes work together—that is, whether or not you have stereoscopic vision.

Some patients choose to leave one eye untreated or to have it only partially corrected, which allows them to read without glasses for a longer period of time. This is called monovision and will be more thoroughly discussed further on. People whose eyes do not naturally work in stereo adjust more quickly to monovision than do people whose eyes work together. Adjustment problems can include fluctuating vision, dizziness, nausea, and headaches. These symptoms are usually mild but nonetheless can be uncomfortable. Some people never adjust. Others have no problem. For example, I opted to leave my left, nondominant eye untreated to achieve monovision. Because my eyes were not naturally stereoscopic prior to treatment, I had absolutely no difficulty adjusting to monovision. For me, it was no big deal.

Dr. Brint adds, "If it turns out that a patient is not happy with monovision, it can be reversed. The surgeon can treat an untreated eye or perform a second procedure on an undercorrected eye."

Many of these tests will be conducted again after you have laser vision correction.

Treatment Decisions

A comprehensive eye examination and a consultation regarding the benefits, risks, and potential complications of laser vision correction will tell you whether you are a good candidate medically. They also will help you decide whether you are certain that you want to permanently alter the shape of your cornea. And they will ensure that you are prepared for anything that might happen during or after the procedure.

However, the decision-making process isn't over yet. You still have to decide how to manage presbyopia if you are nearing or past the age of 40, whether to have PRK or LASIK, and whether to have surgery on both eyes on the same day or different days. Now is also the time to discuss with the doctor your lifestyle, profession, and personal preferences, which will affect the decisions you make about treatment. For example, a professional athlete might make a different choice than someone who spends all day at a desk reading legal briefs on paper or on a computer monitor. If your hobbies require that you see close detail, you might make a different choice than if your hobby is bird watching. Your doctor can help you to discover what choices are available and which ones might work for you.

> *Be advised, if you are near or in your 40s, that even if you are not yet presbyopic, you eventually will be after laser vision correction, just as you would be if you didn't have laser vision correction.*

If you are nearing 40 or older, you already are or will very soon begin to lose the ability to accommodate. It becomes more difficult to adjust your vision from far to near and back again. Eventually, you will lose your near vision. This is called presbyopia, and it happens to all of us. Nearsighted people often can manage presbyopia, at least for a few years, by removing their distance lenses. It's not unusual to see eyeglass-wearing restaurant patrons remove their glasses to read the menu. People with hyperopia, or farsightedness, don't have that advantage. If you wear corrective lenses full-time for near and far vision, then you probably will wear bifocals when you become presbyopic, or you will have a separate pair of glasses for reading. Some hyperopes have trifocals or three pairs of corrective lenses for near, far, and mid-range vision.

Be advised, if you are near or in your 40s, that even if you are not yet presbyopic, you eventually will be after laser vision correction, just as you would be if you didn't have laser vision correction. You will wear reading glasses, and the strength of the lenses needed to read comfortably may change several times during the first few months as your eyes heal. For many "40-something" post–laser vision correction patients, buying inexpensive, over-the-counter glasses purchased at the local pharmacy can keep costs down during the transition phase. Once your vision stabilizes, if you find you need reading glasses, you will want to visit your primary eye-care doctor and make sure you get the right prescription.

Monovision

As mentioned earlier, people who have refractive surgery just before or during the onset of presbyopia can elect to leave one eye untreated or to have one eye partially corrected, which will enable them to continue reading without corrective lenses for quite a long time. Essentially, what you are doing with monovision is using one eye for distance vision and one eye for near vision.

Of course, one of the main reasons people have refractive surgery is to become less dependent on eyeglasses and contact lenses. And if people are perfectly honest, most will tell you that they decided to have refractive surgery hoping to free themselves of corrective eyewear altogether. Therefore, it might be tempting to jump at the monovision option. Don't.

Many people adjust very nicely to monovision. In fact, lots of people have achieved the same results with contact lenses for years by wearing a contact lens in their nondominant eye, which does not fully correct the myopic refractive error. However, monovision compromises your depth perception. If you are a competitive athlete—say, a golfer or a marksman—clear, sharp distance vision is critical. Just as critical is the ability to judge distance. Monovision makes it more difficult to judge distance.

When both eyes work in stereo, light travels through each eye at a slightly different angle, ending up at a single point. It is because light enters the eye from different angles that we are able to know when one object is in front of another and to distinguish that which is far away or traveling toward us. Monovision compromises that ability. For many people that is not a handicap; for some it is. Pilots, for example, would not want to have monovision, nor would race car drivers. In fact, anyone who drives a vehicle for a living probably wouldn't be comfortable with monovision.

It is possible to mimic monovision with contact lenses. If you're interested and you can tolerate contact lenses, ask your doctor to help you simulate monovision with contacts. Also, discuss with your doctor what you hope to achieve by choosing monovision. It may not be the right decision for you, based on your lifestyle, profession, or hobbies.

If you decide to give monovision a try with contact lenses, it's important to realize that a trial of an hour or two won't be enough. You will need a week or more to determine if you can adjust. And even then, contact lenses are not a true test because whenever you are uncomfortable, you can pop them out. Once your vision is permanently corrected, there is nothing you can do but return to the surgeon to have the partially corrected eye fully corrected. Fortunately, that can be done fairly easily.

PRK or LASIK

Early on, this question was a bigger issue than it is now. For one thing, the FDA's Ophthalmic Device Advisory Panel in July 1999 recommended approval of both the VISX and Summit laser for use in LASIK within certain boundaries. For another, most busy refractive surgeons now routinely recommend LASIK. Although a panel recommendation does not guarantee approval, the FDA has a history of following the recommendations of its panels. Because the FDA has approved both lasers for use in LASIK, refractive surgeons who recommend PRK probably do so because of their own lack of experience with the instruments used in

LASIK rather than because they are convinced that PRK is a superior procedure.

Patients with low to moderate refractive errors will achieve good results with either procedure. People with high refractive errors get better results with LASIK. There are advantages and disadvantages to both procedures.

LASIK patients experience very little discomfort, if any, after the procedure. PRK patients can have significant discomfort for 24 to 48 hours. An article published in the April 15, 1999, professional journal *Ocular Surgery News* reported that "The common symptoms of pain, foreign body sensation, burning, and tearing were approximately six times greater in PRK patients versus LASIK patients." Of course, the study included results from just twenty-one patients (ten PRK and eleven LASIK) who were monitored at 2 hours, 5 hours, 24 hours, 48 hours, and 72 hours. It's hard to draw conclusions based on a handful of patients when millions have had laser vision correction.

Anecdotally, Dr. Brint can tell you that of all the patients he has treated, the ones who had PRK spoke more frequently of extreme postoperative discomfort than did those who had LASIK. I can report that I was very uncomfortable for the first 48 hours after PRK; my eyes burned, watered, and felt scratchy. I was extremely photophobic and when traveling home found that constant application of artificial tears did nothing for the symptoms brought on by the dry air in the plane. I simply couldn't keep my eyes open. Two former colleagues of mine, Betsy Osterhout and Joan Reich, who had surgery within a few weeks of my own, also in Canada, had experiences very similar to mine. On the other hand, Drs. Whitten, Rubinfeld, and Kameen, all practicing refractive surgeons in the Washington, D.C., area, also had PRK in Canada prior to FDA approval of the excimer laser for use in PRK. Each doctor expressed that he had no postoperative discomfort. Dr. Whitten played golf within hours of surgery.

Dr. Brint had LASIK and experienced no discomfort. In fact, he was on an airplane four hours after surgery, feeling great.

And, of course, since then, doctors have learned a lot more about the management of discomfort after PRK, and patients are less likely to have to experience such extreme discomfort. Furthermore, even those who had real, significant pain still report that they would have PRK all over again to reduce their dependence on corrective lenses.

LASIK patients see better faster. Doctors call this the WOW factor. With PRK, visual recovery can be weeks, even months, with each day bringing improvement, but with noticeable fluctuations in vision during the course of a day or week. Within twenty-four hours most LASIK patients can see more clearly than they have ever seen before without lenses; they are astounded.

The WOW Factor

I learned the real meaning of the WOW factor when working at the TLC Boca Raton center in Florida with my co-author, Dr. Brint, and optometrist Sal DeCanio, executive director of TLC Boca Raton. I was there to facilitate training of new doctors and to conduct a patient education seminar. As part of the physician training, Dr. Brint performed LASIK on six patients. The next morning all six returned for their first post-op visit. Five had an animated conversation about the wonders of LASIK. None reported pain; all enthusiastically showed off their new visual acuity by holding a hand over first one eye and then the other and reading signs across the lobby. Several embraced Drs. Brint and DeCanio, some with tears of joy in their eyes.

One of the six wasn't interested in joining in. I asked him if everything was all right. And he said, yes, if I meant did he feel okay or was he in pain? He was not in pain. But no, he wasn't all right, in that he was not experiencing the same clarity of vision that the others around him enjoyed. He couldn't understand what all the fuss was about. Drs. Brint and DeCanio quickly escorted him back to the exam room. It turned out that the young man had not been fully corrected. For him, there was no WOW factor. A retreatment fixed the problem, and I'm happy to report that his vision is now 20/20 and he eagerly shares his success story with others.

Both LASIK and PRK patients complain of light sensitivity (also called photophobia), but PRK patients seem to be more sensitive for longer periods of time.

With LASIK there is minimal risk of haze. PRK patients often experience mild, transient haze. Haze occurs during the healing process as new collagen fibers are created. During formation, they can give the cornea a grainy appearance. Haze is detectable in a slit lamp exam, with its high magnification, but generally is not noticed by the patient. Sometimes, though, it can create a problem with glare at night because when bright lights reach the fibers, the rays scatter. Haze is treated with corticosteroidal eyedrops and almost always recedes over time.

Both LASIK and PRK patients complain of light sensitivity (also called photophobia), but PRK patients seem to be more sensitive for longer periods of time.

A very small risk of infection is associated with PRK and LASIK; PRK carries a somewhat greater risk. To accomplish PRK, the surgeon first removes the topmost layer of corneal tissue, called the epithelium, which usually grows back within two to three days. It is an open wound and until the wound heals, there is a risk of infection, however slight, which is decreased by wearing a protective bandage contact lens. The possibility is made even more remote in both procedures by the routine application of antibiotic eyedrops just before and just after treatment. PRK patients also are given antibiotic eyedrops to take at home during the first few days of recovery. Says Dr. Brint, "It is a well-known fact that infection is much more common in contact lens wearers than it is in patients who have PRK or LASIK."

Flap Complications

Arguably, the only real advantage of PRK over LASIK is that in PRK there is no risk of corneal flap complications, because there is no flap. For people who are risk-averse, that could be a big advantage. To complete the LASIK procedure, the surgeon cuts a thin slice of corneal tissue (flap) with a device called a microkeratome. The flap is lifted off the corneal surface, like opening a book, until the laser beam has been applied to the stroma, completing the desired correction. Then the flap is replaced over the treatment area and it adheres naturally, without stitches, to the surface of the eye.

It is in the creation of the flap that problems can occur. If the suction ring that is used to hold the eye steady and to expose the cornea while a pass is made with the microkeratome is jostled, suction can be lost. This can result in an incomplete cap, or the surgeon might end up with a cap that is much too small. Rarely, a defective microkeratome blade results in a ragged-edged cap, which can cause problems later on during healing; or the microkeratome creates a cap without a hinge, called a "free cap." With the newer microkeratomes, free caps are less frequent. Dr. Brint adds that "Free caps are easily managed by experienced surgeons, as LASIK was originally done always with 'free caps,' which were marked for easy alignment."

As long as you have an experienced surgeon, none of these complications are sight-compromising, but the procedure might have to be postponed on that day and you would have to return home to wait for the eye to heal, usually about three months. This is where experience really counts—both in preventing this problem and also in knowing how to properly deal with the situation should it occur. (See chapter 7 for a discussion of side effects and complications associated with laser vision correction.)

There are patients for whom PRK is a safer or more expedient alternative. For the protective corneal flap to be created, the microkeratome must pass unimpeded across the surface of the eye. Some people's eyes are so deep-set that achieving good exposure of the cornea with the microkeratome's suction ring is difficult. Patients with a condition called recurrent corneal erosions, in which the epithelium doesn't want to stay "stuck down," are believed to be better candidates for PRK than for LASIK. People with thin corneas and moderate to high refractive errors are candidates for PRK but perhaps not for LASIK.

Adds Dr. Kennedy, "Remember, as was just mentioned, there are certain ocular conditions where PRK may be the best choice for you. Keep an open mind: just because there are numerous advantages to LASIK, doesn't mean PRK isn't a good choice for you, depending on your circumstances. Your doctor can advise you."

If you've done your homework and have found an experienced surgeon who works with an experienced laser vision correction team, virtually any situation that arises in the laser suite can be managed and will not affect your long-term visual results. So the decision whether to have PRK or LASIK should be made by you and your doctor; however, you can be certain that most surgeons and most laser centers will recommend, and maybe even encourage, LASIK.

One Eye at a Time or Both on the Same Day?

Whether to have both eyes treated on the same day or to have first one eye treated and then the second procedure performed several days, a week, or even a few months later is less of an issue than it once was.

When the excimer laser was approved by the FDA for use in PRK, the treatment guidelines issued by the agency to the laser's manufacturers included communicating with surgeons that they should treat one eye at a time and wait a full three months before treating the second eye. The reason those instructions were included as part of the approval was because this was the procedure during the clinical trials.

Before a medical device is approved for use in the United States, its manufacturer must undertake rigorous, supervised testing. This is called a clinical trial. In order to begin clinical trials, the manufacturer must submit to the FDA an application that includes exactly which tests will be conducted, by whom, and under what conditions. This is called the treatment protocol. (See chapter 10 for a more detailed discussion of the FDA approval process.)

Because doctors were learning about human healing responses after laser surgery, it was determined that a person's eyes should be treated at least three months apart. At the time it was a cautious step, as not enough was known about healing patterns and visual recovery. Furthermore, no two people heal exactly alike, and each of a person's eyes can heal slightly differently. The safer course was to treat first one eye, wait a significant period of time to learn how the patient would respond, and then treat the second eye. Today, of course, surgeons know a great deal more about how the laser affects corneal tissue and about the infinite variety of healing responses and, therefore, are better equipped to manage all patients postoperatively.

Another reason why many surgeons in the early days recommended a three-month waiting period between procedures is that their malpractice insurance companies insisted on following the FDA recommended treatment protocol. Since then, most insurance companies have lifted that restriction.

Do some surgeons still believe it's a good idea to wait at least a day or two between procedures? Yes. Some surgeons would say that in their ideal world, where the only consideration is to do what is medically most conservative, they would want patients to wait at least a day, and even better a week, between procedures. Just in case.

> *Some surgeons would say that in their ideal world, where the only consideration is to do what is medically most conservative, they would want patients to wait at least a day, and even better a week, between procedures. Just in case.*

However, the vast majority of patients would prefer to go once, have both eyes treated, go back to work, and get on with life. Simultaneous bilateral procedures (treating both eyes on the same day) are a patient-driven phenomenon. Early adopters, those who had the procedure before the laser was approved in the United States or just after, often traveled great distances to have their vision corrected. They weren't about to make the journey twice. Fairly quickly, bilateral procedures became routine. Now, it's difficult to find a surgeon who doesn't expect to do both eyes on the same day.

Notes Dr. Brint, "Studies at Emory University and by Dr. Howard Gimbel in Canada, have shown that in thousands of cases, the risk of treating both eyes at the same time was no greater than treating one eye at a time."

So, if you're ready, make your plans and read on. In the next chapter we will tell you what to expect on the day of surgery, as well as in the days, weeks, and months afterward.

6

What Can I Expect?

Congratulations! You have reached one of the most important decisions you will ever make. Certainly, reducing your dependence on eyeglasses and contact lenses might improve the quality of your life, no matter what your current level of vision. Think about all the times you've made a midnight dash to the store for contact lens solution or fumbled around for your glasses on the bedside table. How many times have your glasses fogged over when coming in after a run on a cold day? How many contacts have you lost or pairs of eyeglasses have you broken? Laser vision correction can't guarantee that you will never experience any of those problems again, but in most cases it will reduce your dependence on corrective lenses.

Now that you've made this big decision, there almost certainly will be people around you—coworkers, family members, even your spouse—who will ask: Are you crazy? The answer is no, you're not crazy.

You're not crazy if you decide to have the surgery, and you're not crazy if you decide it's not right for you. This is a very personal decision and you shouldn't let anyone talk you into it or out of it unless it's discovered that you are medically unsuited for refractive surgery. People who have never depended on contact lenses or eyeglasses for good vision have no idea how handicapped someone feels when he or she must rely on corrective lenses for the simplest of tasks. Things that the "normally" sighted take for granted, like reading the alarm clock when first waking up or navigating to the bathroom in the middle of the night, are challenging for people with poor vision. Fear is a constant companion when you can't recognize even familiar faces from more than a few feet away and when, without your lenses, you couldn't in an emergency find your own child in a swimming pool, lake, or ocean.

This is a very personal decision and you shouldn't let anyone talk you into it or out of it unless it's discovered that you are medically unsuited for refractive surgery.

In the introduction, I wrote about the Washington, D.C., doctor's wife who was adamantly opposed to her husband having laser vision correction. She was until his doctor, Dr. Rubinfeld, showed her what the world looked like to her husband by putting in front of her eyes lenses that produced the same blurry vision that he had. She immediately gave her consent. If your spouse, partner, or parent is equally adamant in his or her opposition, bring that person with you to your preoperative appointment or to the center on the day of surgery and ask the doctor or technician to replicate your vision for them with a lens. It will make a world of difference in their appreciation of your situation. They might even stop asking you if you're crazy.

Laura Pratt, a reporter for the *National Post* in Canada, wrote an article about her experience undergoing LASIK. In an effort to explain why she, who describes herself as fearful, and whom her surgeon, Dr. Jeffery Machat, described to me as more than a little skeptical, would allow a virtual stranger to tamper with "this most precious body part," she wrote the following:

> I relished the thought of being able to see the alarm clock in the wee hours of the morning, to enjoy a bath without fogging up my glasses, to open my eyes and see the lake when I go swimming. And I could also relate to the 'Why I did it' tales Dr. Machat shared in his office that day. The woman who was asked to remove her glasses in preparation for an emergency airplane landing, who promised herself she'd have the surgery if she survived the experience. The man who lost track of his family on vacation when a strong undercurrent pushed his lens-less self way down the beach during a swim. The woman who rested her glasses on the deck of the pool, then panicked when one of her kids swam out of her field of vision.
>
> "But there was something more that propelled me into this terrifying place (specifically: prone, under a blade that was about to sunder through the top layer of my eye). It was, I think, an act of rebellion against my aging self. A rally against the erosion of what I had always understood to be a lifelong gift. It was Dylan Thomas–like terrorism against my own dying light. Other people get facelifts; I got a vision lift.

There are myriad life-enhancing reasons why people with poor vision would want to reduce their dependence on corrective lenses. When I began research for this book, I invited all of the TLC centers to submit patient stories, testimonials, and patient letters to provide background and color for the book. I received a flood of e-mail, phone calls, and "snail mail." All were delightful accounts of just how extraordinary a change it is to no longer be dependent on corrective lenses. Even many patients whose recovery was challenging as a result of complications or temporary surgical side effects insisted they would do it all over again.

Dr. Brint and Dr. Kennedy have had countless conversations with patients who are amazed at how much sharper and brighter everything looks when seen without corrective lenses.

In my interviews and in their interactions with patients, the most commonly used word to describe the postoperative results was *miracle*. The postoperative euphoria many feel is described as excitement, joy, wonder, and astonishment. More astonishing, however, are some of the patients who elect to have the procedure. Robert Hall, center manager for TLC Tri-Cities, wrote the following in response to my request for patient stories:

Over the past several years, I have seen many moving sights with patients' families and friends at the viewing window as their loved ones underwent laser vision correction. I've held back tears on more than one occasion. Perhaps the most moving experience was when one of our patients, a tetraplegic, came in for surgery.

This patient had lost his mobility many years before in an accident, which left him with only limited use of his hands and arms. He wanted to have laser vision correction because he had so much trouble dealing with eyeglasses on a daily basis and there was no way he could wear contact lenses. Instead of being angry and bitter, he had one of the most positive attitudes of anyone I had ever encountered, regardless of physical condition.

The center asked two emergency medical technicians (EMTs) from a nearby station to come on the day of surgery to ensure that the patient was lifted properly from his wheelchair to the laser bed and back again. I stood at the viewing window with the patient's brother, explaining the procedure step by step. The surgery went smoothly. Typically, as soon as the surgery is over we invite our patients to sit up on the laser bed and ask them if they can see the clock on the wall, which is about ten feet away. They almost always can, and they often are amazed. In this patient's case, we were more concerned about return-ing him safely to his wheelchair than about impressing him with his new vision.

Much to my amazement, as the EMTs lifted him into his chair, he looked at the wall, saw the clock, and, gathering what seemed to be all the energy he could muster, turned toward his brother and me and gave us a 'thumbs up.' I had to swallow the lump in my throat and hold back the tears. With all this man had been through over the years, we had been able to help him eliminate one of his handicaps and to improve the quality of his life in a significant way.

Whatever your reason, it's your reason. Only you know the value to you of life with fewer vision-related obstacles. But remember, the surgery, like any surgery, involves accepting a certain amount of risk.

Informed Consent

At some time during the decision-making process, proba-bly right before you have the procedure, someone may tell you a horrifying story of a person who had his or her vision surgically corrected and now can hardly see. Dr. Brint knows from experience that most of these "horror stories" are exaggerated. Often they are about a patient who went from 20/600 to 20/25 instead of 20/20.

If you're a women who's had a baby, it's a little bit like when you're pregnant and people can't wait to tell you hor-ror stories of thirty-six-hour labors, endless agony, and col-icky babies when it's all over.

You can be assured that no one has ever been left per-manently blind as a result of laser vision correction. Some people have had complications that caused serious prob-lems during recovery, and a very few have vision worse than it was before the surgery. A very small percentage of patients have lost lines of vision, which means their best corrected visual acuity (BCVA) (see chapter 5 for an explanation of BCVA) is not as good after the surgery as it was before the surgery.

Of course, it could be that your BCVA before surgery was 20/15 or even 20/10 (some people who wear rigid gas-permeable lenses are correctable to better than 20/20) and after surgery your BCVA is 20/20. Your surgically corrected vision is excellent, but it is still not as good as it was when wearing contact lenses. Most people can live with the change, but not everyone. And there are patients whose BCVA was 20/20 prior to surgery and is 20/30 or 20/40 after surgery. Again, 20/30 is good vision and will allow for an unrestricted driver's license in every state, but it isn't 20/20. For most tasks 20/30 is good enough, but some patients would still want very thin spectacle lenses for activities such as night driving. Furthermore, if the surgeon deems it advisable, an enhancement also could be performed to achieve 20/20.

These are among the risks your doctor and/or the staff of the laser center where you plan to have your procedure should already have discussed with you. If they have not by this point, they will before you have surgery.

Preferably during the preoperative consultation or perhaps a few days prior to surgery, you will be asked to read and sign a document called an informed consent. Some doctors and some laser centers will not ask you to read and sign the document until the day of surgery. It's a better idea to read the informed consent ahead of time, in your own doctor's office or at home, as long as there is a contact number and a person you can call with questions.

Some doctors are reluctant to present you with this choice because they are concerned that the language used to describe associated risks and complications will frighten you enough to cancel surgery. But it isn't a good idea to wait until the day of surgery to read the document because you are bound to be nervous about the surgery anyway and that nervousness may make it more difficult for you to fully understand the risks associated with laser vision correction. Dr. Brint adds that it also isn't a good idea to read it without having someone available who completely understands the procedure, to clarify the inevitable questions you will have.

> *You can be assured that no one has ever been left permanently blind as a result of laser vision correction.*

And as Dr. Mark Whitten points out: "If it turns out that after reading the informed consent patients are too frightened to have surgery, then you don't really want those patients in the laser room anyway because they're not ready to live with their decision. They're the patients who come back time and time again with various visual complaints that can't be substantiated by an eye exam. But their symptoms are very real, and they are undoubtedly sorry they ever had the procedure. That's not good for them, and it's not good for the reputation of the doctor or the laser center where the patient was treated."

If you have decided to have laser vision correction, have made an appointment for surgery, and have not yet seen an informed consent document, don't be shy. Call your doctor or the center where the procedure will be performed. Ask them to send you a copy of the informed consent. Read it carefully. You probably will have questions about the risks (the scary part). Write them down so you can call to have them answered, or bring them with you on the day of surgery. Be sure that all of your questions are answered to your satisfaction before you sign the document, which must be signed by you and the surgeon in the presence of witnesses.

If you've ever had surgery of any kind as an adult, then you've signed an informed consent. It's a document that tells you every possible thing that could go wrong during or after the surgery and requires that you affirm by your signature that those risks have been described to you and that you understand what has been said.

There is no informed consent template, no central organization that drafts and distributes such documents. However, associations such as the American Optometric Association (AOA), the American Academy of Ophthalmology (AAO), and the American Society of Cataract and Refractive Surgeons (ASCRS) do have sample documents that doctors can customize for their own use. All laser-center management companies have attorneys draft such documents, each of which looks slightly different and uses somewhat different language to describe the procedure and its associated risks.

TLC's informed consent document, which is distributed to its network of 11,000 doctors, is nearly ten pages long and requires that the patient and a witness initial each paragraph. Patients also are required to rewrite an exact copy of certain phrases in the document, such as "I may not achieve the result I hope for" and "I may still need to wear glasses," to ensure that the patient has read, heard, and understood each caution. It's a most intimidating document, but once you pass that hurdle, the rest is smooth sailing.

The Process Begins—Arriving at the Center

On the day of your procedure, you need to arrive at the laser center at least one hour prior to your scheduled laser time. Some centers ask that you arrive as early as two hours before surgery. You will remain in your street clothes for the procedure, so think comfort. "And warmth," says Dr. Brint. "The laser rooms are usually cold because the laser works better in those conditions." Loose-fitting clothing is a good idea. Many laser centers ask that you refrain from wearing cologne or perfume, as the fumes can damage the laser's delicate optics (mirrors that direct the laser beam). For the same reason, centers don't allow harsh cleaning fluids to be used in the laser room.

Obviously, you won't want to wear eye makeup and because some centers ask you to remove earrings before surgery, you might just want to go without. Leave your pager and cell phone out of the laser suite, too. If they go off, the sound might distract you and the surgeon.

Expect to feel a mixture of anxiety and excitement. You may even briefly wonder whether you should go through with it. Don't be concerned; mixed emotions are perfectly normal. Fortunately, you will be in the company of people who really do know how you feel, as they've helped many patients through the process. Furthermore, many laser-center staff members and surgeons have had their own vision corrected and are well able to empathize. They are prepared to calm your fears and to answer any last-minute questions. Many people in the reception area will probably be going through the very same thing as you. The environment often is quite collegial.

Even those of us who are in the industry and who have watched hundreds of procedures are still nervous when the eyes being treated are our own. For example, Betsy Osterhout, executive director of TLC Mt. Laurel (New Jersey), had PRK in Canada in 1996. She is a registered nurse and had been a sales representative for ophthalmic device and product companies for years. In her career, she has watched hundreds of surgeons perform thousands of cataract surgeries, and by the time she had her procedure, she had watched hundreds of excimer laser treatments. Yet she was anxious, nonetheless, when the day of her surgery arrived.

As Betsy tells the story: "I remember still being very nervous, even though I had seen a lot of procedures done in Canada. It was terrifying for me. I knew that I had made the right decision, but I can remember thinking to myself, 'What have I done, have I lost my mind?' Because as much as I was educated, and as many procedures as I had seen, I still felt at that moment that I would be the one, that I would lose my vision and that would be the end of my world. So, I did have that fear, even though I also had confidence. And, of course, my husband didn't help because he kept asking, 'Are you sure?' And my mother and father thought I was a little bit crazy, especially because I had to go all the way to Canada."

The truth is, your nervousness can help you to remain alert and to pay closer attention to any directions given you by the surgeon in the laser room.

Bring Your Partner or Friend

You are welcome and encouraged to bring your spouse, your partner, a friend, or a family member to the center and to have them remain with you as you go through the process. In any case, you must arrange for someone to pick you up after the procedure. If you can't arrange a ride, be sure to let the receptionist at the laser center know that. Generally, the center is prepared to make such arrangements with a taxi or shuttle service. Although you probably will feel fine when you leave, driving yourself is not a good idea. For one thing, your vision may be foggy for the first few hours; for another, the anesthesia will begin to wear off and your eyes will feel a little scratchy and you might have a burning sensation.

When you arrive, you may sign in just as you would in any doctor's office and take a seat in the reception area. There, a patient consultant will greet you and escort you to an office where your file will be reviewed to ensure that all the paperwork is in order, including the informed consent discussed earlier. If you have not already paid, you will be asked for payment at this time. Many centers and many physicians do offer flexible payment programs; however, those need to be worked out prior to the day of surgery. (See chapter 9 for a discussion of the business of laser vision correction.)

Although you probably will feel fine when you leave, driving yourself is not a good idea.

Once payment has been made, you will be escorted to a preoperative waiting area. At this time, some patients are asked to repeat certain tests that already have been done during the preoperative examination by their doctor or at the laser center. Sometimes the surgeon will ask for a corneal topography on the day of the surgery, to compare it with previous maps to make absolutely certain of the treatment plan. If your doctor did not take a pachymeter reading (which measures the thickness of your cornea), the surgeon will ask that the measurement be performed at this time.

Who administers these tests depends on who is available. For example, a patient consultant often does the topography, although a pachymetry reading is more likely to be handled by an ophthalmic technician or the surgeon.

About fifteen to twenty minutes prior to surgery you probably will be escorted to an exam lane, where a technician or an optometrist might give you another manifest refraction. Again, this depends on whether or not the surgeon is 100 percent comfortable with the numbers he or she is about to have the technician program into the laser.

Here, patients will meet with their surgeons. Some will see the same surgeon they visited for their pre-op exam, but it is not at all uncommon for patients to meet their surgeons for the first time at the laser center on the day of surgery.

This is particularly true for surgeons who frequently co-manage patients with the same primary eye-care doctor.

For example, in the Washington, D.C., area, ophthalmologist Mark Whitten and optometrist Harry Snyder have successfully co-managed hundreds of patients. Dr. Snyder's patients are confident in his recommendation. They trust the referral to Dr. Whitten, who has performed tens of thousands of procedures. Aware of his reputation, most patients don't ask to meet with Dr. Whitten prior to the day of surgery.

There are many such co-management teams around the country. For example, Dr. Kameen frequently co-manages with optometrists Jamie Hess and Rob Leikin. And Dr. Brint works with Dr. Lori Blackmer in Mississippi, who also had the procedure. Comments Dr. Brint, "She knows the patient's visual/optical history much better than I could, has had her patient out of contact lenses an appropriate length of time, and checks for the stability of the refractive prescription, which is crucial. She also has had plenty of time to discuss the procedure and answer any questions. By the time the patients make the fifty-mile trip to New Orleans, they are ready to meet me, go ahead with the surgery, make the trip home, and see her for the postoperative care, knowing that she is completely trained in recognizing any postoperative problems, not just the more common ones such as temporary dry eyes. She also knows when a problem requires my attention and that I am only a phone call away."

While in the exam room, also called an exam lane, the surgeon will meet with you briefly and answer any last-minute questions. If a technician or patient consultant has not already applied the first set of eyedrops—one to anesthetize the cornea, one to prevent infection, and a third to control postoperative inflammation—the surgeon might do so at this time, if it is within five minutes or so of your procedure. The surgeon usually receives your patient file from the co-managing doctor or from the center where your pre-operative exam was conducted as much as a week before surgery; however, sometimes the file arrives only the day before. If the surgeon has any questions at all, he or she might ask that certain tests be repeated, such as a double-check of your refractive prescription, and might decide to do a quick exam to satisfy any lingering doubts or concerns about the desired correction.

This also is your opportunity to ask the surgeon any last-minute questions. It is not the time to discuss treatment decisions, such as PRK or LASIK or whether to try mono-vision, although I have been with doctors just before sur-gery when patients have raised those questions. (See chapter 5 for a discussion of treatment decisions.) Decisions that are so critical to good care and a positive outcome need to be made long before you are about to have surgery.

While in the exam lane, or perhaps even before when you first meet with the patient consultant, you will be given postoperative instructions. Most centers also will give you a postoperative kit that contains the eyedrops you will need for the next several days—longer if you have PRK. These include an anti-inflammatory drop to reduce postop-erative swelling, antibiotic eyedrops if you've had PRK, and artificial tears, which are used to keep your eyes moist. The kit probably also will contain an over-the-counter pain medication such as Tylenol or Advil, wraparound sun-glasses, eye shields for use at night, and instructions and a telephone number to call in an emergency.

Listen carefully to any postoperative instructions given. Generally, they will be to go home and take a nap. Sleep will aid the healing process, and very likely you will be tired emotionally and physically because the adrenaline rush will be over. And, most important of all, you will be instructed not to rub your eyes.

Once you have spoken with the surgeon, you will be escorted to a patient waiting area just outside the laser room. Many centers have observation areas and invite patients and partners to watch procedures while they wait for their turn in the laser room.

Let me caution you, if you didn't like the video, you won't like it any better live on a large TV monitor. Only you know your tolerance for such "real life" observation. There is no blood, so you don't have to be squeamish about that, but you will see the surgeon pass the micro-keratome over the cornea, slide a thin metal instrument under the flap, lift the flap, and flip it over. And for some people, seeing a patient on the laser bed and watching as the surgeon does that first pass makes it all a little too real. They would rather know without seeing. I've talked with lots of patients who couldn't bring themselves to watch a live procedure until afterward. Others watch cheerfully and just as cheerfully enter the laser room for their own procedures.

While you are waiting, you may receive a second set of eyedrops, all for the same purpose as the first set, and you may be asked to put on a disposable surgical "bonnet." This varies by laser center and by surgeon. The bonnet keeps your hair out of the way, and it also helps to keep the laser room clean. It is not necessary to perform refractive surgery in a completely sterile environment to avoid infection, but extraordinary efforts are taken to minimize the amount of contaminants in the air, as they can damage the laser's optics. Infection is a risk of refractive surgery but a minimal one, so the lack of a completely sterile environment is not a cause for concern.

Some surgeons and some centers routinely offer patients a mild sedative, such as Valium, as much to help patients sleep after the procedure as to calm their nerves during surgery. Using a sedative is up to you and your doctor, but most patients don't find it necessary. And almost all say afterward that being completely alert during surgery helped them to follow the surgeon's instructions.

In the Laser Room

When it is your "turn," you will be escorted into the laser room by a patient consultant or a technician. This person will guide you to the laser bed (which really looks more like a dentist's chair but is called a bed nonetheless) and will ask you to lie down. The bed pivots. When you've been made comfortable, someone will swing the laser bed under the laser. You will be staring directly into the laser's operating microscope, in which there is a red or green light, depending on which laser is used.

There will be three or four other people in the laser room when you enter. One is the laser technician who is responsible for programming and operating the laser under the surgeon's supervision. Another technician hands to the surgeon items used during surgery, and assembles and disassembles the microkeratome. A third might prepare equipment for sterilization, escort patients in and out of the laser room, set up for the next patient, and/or perform other chores that ensure efficient delivery of patient care.

> *When you've been made comfortable, someone will swing the laser bed under the laser. You will be staring directly into the laser's operating microscope, in which there is a red or green light, depending on which laser is used.*

Before reclining, look around. Mainly, what you will see is the laser, as it takes up most of the space in the room. Right next to the laser, to the left of the laser bed and within reach of the surgeon's stool, will be a metal stand covered in a white or sometimes blue cloth. On it will be everything the surgeon will need during surgery, except the microkeratome, which often is behind the surgeon on a counter or table. Generally, the cart contains:

- Three bottles of eyedrops: anesthetic, antibiotic, and anti-inflammatory
- A pad containing water-soluble ink for marking the cornea, to ensure proper repositioning of the flap upon completion of the procedure
- An eyelid speculum, used to help hold your eyelids open
- An irrigation "squirter," a syringe-like tool containing sterile saline solution, which will be used to flood the area around the suction ring just before the microkeratome pass and after the flap has been repositioned
- A slim metal instrument called an optical zone or LASIK marker, used to mark the area of the cornea where the flap will be created
- A thin metal instrument called a spatula, used to lift the corneal flap
- A tonometer (plastic cone-shaped device), which is used to ensure that adequate pressure has been achieved prior to the microkeratome pass
- Little white sponges on a blue stick, called Merocel sponges

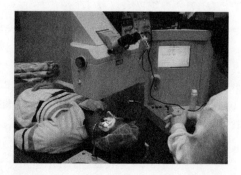

A patient undergoing laser vision correction.

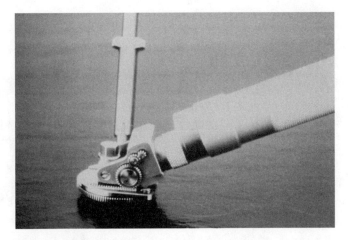

The microkeratome.

On a counter or table behind the surgeon you might see the microkeratome and the black power pack to which it is attached by a tube. The power pack creates the suction that grasps the cornea by the suction ring, to ensure the best possible exposure of the cornea for an accurate, clean cut.

Any other equipment you see will depend on where you have the surgery. In some laser rooms there is a microscope on a counter just behind where the surgeon sits, which is used to check the microkeratome blade before use. Other laser rooms have dehumidifiers to maintain a constant level of humidity, and some have emergency exhaust systems to expel gas from the room in the event of a leak. And as in every other doctor's office, there might be counters filled with supplies used during the procedure.

Preparations for Surgery

Once you are comfortably reclining on the laser bed, the surgeon will position himself or herself directly behind you on a stool. If you are having bilateral surgery (which means both eyes will be treated on the same day), the eye to be treated second will be patched. The other eye will be prepared for surgery. Some surgeons use a surgical drape to cover the eyelids and to keep eyelashes and other debris away from the cornea and out of the way of the microkeratome. Others tape the eyelashes back away from the corneal surface for the same reason. Still others leave the lashes untouched.

At this point, the surgeon may apply another set of eyedrops. Next, an eyelid speculum will be inserted to help hold your eyelids apart. As bad as this may sound, the speculum doesn't hurt. Some people feel the pressure of the wire against their eyelids and say that it's a little odd at first to be unable to blink but not particularly uncomfortable.

With your eye exposed, you will be asked to stare up into the laser microscope at a blinking red or green light, depending on which laser is used. A circle of light surrounds the blinking light. The surgeon will ask if you can see the light. He or she also will tell you that when instructed to do so, you must fixate on that light, that you are not to move your eyes or your head but must stare at the light.

Throughout the procedure you will be cautioned not to move, but a little movement will not affect the outcome. Furthermore, the surgeon is in complete control of the laser. If for some reason you do move your eyes so that there is concern for the outcome of the surgery, the doctor will simply stop the procedure. When you have been repositioned and reassured, the computer-controlled laser will begin precisely where it left off.

During this interval the laser technician will be "arming" the laser, getting it ready for use by filling the laser's cavity with the mixture of Argon and Fluoride gases used in an excimer laser to create the "lasing effect," that is, produce the laser beam. The technician also will test the laser's energy output, or fluence. You will hear a repetitive noise that is described variously as a snapping, popping, or clicking sound.

You will hear that same sound when the laser is in use during treatment. Most likely, your correction already has been programmed into the laser, as this can be done ahead of time. But at this point the key card will be inserted into the laser. The key card contains information about your treatment. Think of it as a customized computer program with instructions on how many laser pulses will be needed to achieve the desired correction.

The card is also like a credit card, in that it is the means by which laser companies ensure they receive royalty fees for use of the laser. You may have heard of this; it's called the Pillar Point fee. Pillar Point is a patent-protection partnership between VISX Inc. and Summit Technology, to which anyone who uses the laser must pay a $250-per-use fee. This is a controversial issue, too complex to discuss in great detail.

The technician and the surgeon will check the refractive numbers programmed into the laser's computer one last time as a fail-safe. While the laser technician prepares the laser, the surgeon checks the microkeratome, which probably was assembled by another technician. Some surgeons assemble the microkeratome themselves, but most expert surgeons who do large volumes of procedures do not. The surgeon will check the blade for defects, test the suction ring to make certain that adequate vacuum pressure can be achieved, and check the smoothness of the microkeratome's gears. You will hear a whirring sound when the surgeon tests the vacuum pressure and a humming noise as he or she checks the movement of the gears.

The microkeratome pass that creates the thin corneal flap takes only seconds, but it is the most critical step in the process. Improper assembly, gears not meshing smoothly, or inadequate pressure all have potentially serious consequences for the patient. You may be anxious to get the whole thing over with, but be glad that the surgeon and technicians take every precaution in preparation for your ten-minute procedure.

The Procedure Begins

When the surgeon and the technician are certain everything is in working order and the laser's computer has been properly programmed for your treatment, the procedure begins. The surgeon or one of the technicians will talk to you throughout the entire procedure. You will not be left guessing as to what's about to happen.

- The surgeon first will mark your cornea with the optical zone or LASIK marker, making a slight transient indentation in your cornea where the flap will be made.

- A "hatch" mark is placed at two points around the circle (some surgeons use circles as marks), to ensure proper replacement of the flap when the procedure is finished.

- While the surgeon is marking the cornea, you will be able to see his or her hand passing over your eye, but it may look fuzzy or as if you are looking up through water.

- The suction ring is placed on the sclera surrounding the cornea. Care is taken by the surgeon to place the ring directly in the center, slightly to the left or slightly to the right. The surgeon thinks in terms of temporally (toward the temple) or nasally (toward the nose), depending on the treatment plan. This is one of the many decisions surgeons must make to ensure that each treatment gives the best possible results. Dr. Brint adds, "The same principle applies when a different microkeratome, which makes the hinge of the flap above rather than nasally, is used."

- The surgeon will ask for suction. A technician will step on or hit the pedal that activates the microkeratome's suction function; you will hear the same whirring sound you heard when the instrument was being tested.

- When suction is applied, you will not be able to see. Your vision will slowly dim or be completely dark. This will last only seconds, as the microkeratome passes over your cornea and back again.

- Pressure will be tested by touching the cornea with a little, clear plastic cylindrical device called a tonometer.

- Just before the microkeratome is guided across the cornea, the surgeon will use a "squirter" bulb to squirt sterile saline solution into the middle of the suction ring to lubricate the corneal surface.

- With the ring in place, the microkeratome head is placed in the gear tracks of the suction ring. You might feel the surgeon wiggle the instrument while in the ring to make sure that the device is properly inserted. Again, you might feel the movement, but you will not feel pain.

- The surgeon next guides the microkeratome across the track of the suction ring to create the corneal flap, stopping just short of a complete pass, leaving a hinge of tissue prior to reversing the device. Newer microkeratomes have a fixed stopper that prevents them from traveling completely across the cornea, greatly diminishing the risk of what is called a "free cap," or a corneal flap without its hinge. Highly experienced surgeons are not overly concerned about free caps. If it is a clean pass and the cap is of adequate thickness, they simply complete the procedure and put the flap back in place just as they would if there were a hinge. If not, the surgeon stops the procedure, repairs the cap, and the patient goes home to heal, usually returning in

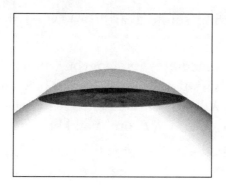

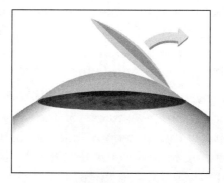

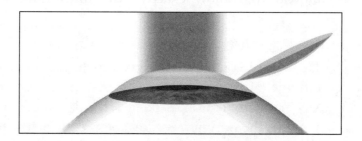

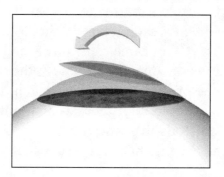

The eye during laser vision correction.

about three months to proceed with the surgery. (See chapter 7 for a complete discussion of risks and complications.)

- When the flap has been created, the suction ring is lifted off the sclera.

- A spatula is slipped under the flap to lift it up slightly and to move it to the side, exposing the inner cornea, called the stroma.

- The laser is engaged and the energy beam applied to the stroma. Most patient education material will tell you that the laser beam can't be seen, but many patients say they can see a very pale blue light ray.

- It is now that you will again hear the popping or clicking of the excimer laser.

- Within thirty to sixty seconds, depending on the amount of correction needed, the laser will stop. While the laser is ablating (vaporizing) the corneal tissue, the laser technician will count down for you, so you will know exactly how much time has elapsed and how much more to go.

- When the laser stops, the surgeon will replace the corneal flap back over the exposed stroma. The first eye is now corrected.

- The bulb-like irrigator tool will again be used to squirt saline solution under the cap to rid the area of any debris and to ensure a smooth surface for the flap to "float" back into place.

- A Merocel sponge will then be used to wipe across the cornea. This will smooth any wrinkles in the corneal flap and will ensure that the cap is properly in place.

- For the next few minutes, you will remain still. If you are having bilateral surgery, the surgeon and technicians will prepare for your second procedure.

- When the second eye is finished, you will be asked to sit up and the doctor or a technician will help you off the laser bed and out of the laser room.
- Almost always there will be a clock on the wall and the surgeon will ask you to look at the clock. You will be able to see the numbers and the hands of the clock, maybe for the first time in your life, but don't expect to see them with crystal clarity. You won't. In fact, it will look a little like someone has taken Vaseline and rubbed it on your eyeglasses. But every hour for the next twenty-four, your vision will become more and more clear.

Post-Operative Period

When your procedure is complete you will be escorted out of the laser room and into the patient waiting area, where you will remain for fifteen or twenty minutes to rest and await the first "flap check" and you will be instructed to rest and keep your eyes closed.

This is more important than you might think, because you probably will feel fine, maybe a little drained from the tension, but otherwise fine and able to move around. I felt wonderful after my procedure, and I did move around—too much, as it turns out. Eleven doctors in training looked at my cornea and asked questions about the experience. After about twenty minutes I felt light-headed and nauseous and very nearly fainted. So, take my advice and the advice of the laser center staff and sit quietly while you wait for the surgeon or staff optometrist to check your flaps.

- After about twenty minutes you will be escorted into the exam room, where the surgeon or a staff optometrist will look at your cornea through the slit lamp to make sure the flap is in place.

- The doctor will again review your postoperative instructions, which generally include taking a nap and using an over-the-counter pain medication for any discomfort. You will be warned that you may be photophobic (light-sensitive) for a few days and that wearing sunglasses whenever you are in bright light, inside and out, is a good idea. Some doctors also recommend that you sleep with eye shields on for the first few nights, so that you don't inadvertently rub your cornea and create wrinkles in the flap.

- You will be instructed how often to use the antibiotics and anti-inflammatory eyedrops and the artificial tears. An immediate side effect of laser vision correction is extremely dry eyes. You will find that you need to use a lot of artificial tears over the next few days and maybe the next few weeks.

- The most important instruction you will be given is to keep your hands away from your eyes. *Do not rub your eyes.* The corneal flap begins to adhere immediately, but a strong enough force can dislodge the flap. It's a good rule to just keep your hands away from your eyes.

- After receiving your instructions and an appointment for your first postoperative exam the next day, you are free to go home. The post-op exam will be in your doctor's office, in the surgeon's office, or at the laser center, depending on your particular situation and needs. Be sure to have that appointment set before you leave the center.

- Have your spouse, partner, or designated other drive you directly home.

- By the time you arrive home, the anesthetic eyedrops will have worn off and your eyes will probably feel scratchy or burny and teary for two to three hours. Some people describe it as feeling rough, like sandpaper under your eyelid; others say it feels like you have grit or an eyelash in your eye. Some say it feels the same as when you have left your contact lenses in too long. Suffice it to say, most people feel some discomfort.

- Many people find that just lying quietly in a darkened room is soothing.

- If it is needed, take Tylenol or Advil and then take a nap. Napping is important. Sleep helps the healing process and gets you through the three or four hours of discomfort. Upon waking, you will notice that your vision already is beginning to clear up and you probably will no longer have the scratchy, uncomfortable feeling, but you might. Don't worry if you do; everyone heals at his or her own pace.

- Within twenty-four hours, your vision should be significantly clearer. You will see better than you have in years. However, do not be surprised if your vision is not crystal clear at this point and if it fluctuates over the next few days and weeks. This is perfectly normal.

- On day one, you will have your first postoperative visit. The doctor will check the flap to ensure that it is still in place and that there are no wrinkles or rough, jagged edges, both of which could lead to problems later. He or she also is checking for debris under the flap and for any signs of infection. There should not be, as you were given antibiotic eyedrops preoperatively and intraoperatively (during surgery).

- You probably will be asked to return for postoperative exams after one week, one month, three months, six months, and one year, and then to return every year thereafter for a routine eye exam.

Of course, if at any time in-between you have a problem with your vision, call the doctor at once. Many small problems that occur after refractive surgery are easily managed. If left untreated, however, serious problems can result. Don't be shy. And don't rely on the advice of friends and family. If you think there is a problem, there might be. Make an appointment and go see the doctor. This is another reason why it's important to be treated by a doctor with lots of refractive experience. If a problem does occur, he or she knows how to fix it.

> *Many small problems that occur after refractive surgery are easily managed. If left untreated, however, serious problems can result.*

Don't be frightened by these cautionary words, and don't worry that you might have a problem and not find out about it until it's too late. That's very unlikely. If, for example, the corneal flap becomes dislodged, you'll know. The pain will be considerable and your vision will be very blurry. Similarly, if your eye is infected, you'll know, because it will be red, swollen, and painful. And remember, infection is very rare in refractive surgery.

Activity Restrictions

Thursday and Friday are the most popular days on which to have refractive surgery, for the obvious reason that the patient then has the weekend to recover, missing just one day of work. But lots of people have the surgery on a Monday, Tuesday, or Wednesday and return to work the very next day. The fact is, no one can tell you exactly how long it will take for you to recover, as everyone experiences the procedure differently and everyone recovers at his or her own pace. Generally speaking, within one to three days you will be able to work, drive, and engage in most normal activities.

Most doctors will tell that you can do all of your usual activities as long as you are able. There are some common-sense guidelines, including:

- Wait one full day before taking a shower. It isn't likely, but a strong-enough water flow could dislodge the cap and if you got shampoo in your eye, it would sting and you would be sorely tempted to rub your eyes. Don't rub your eyes.

- Resume driving when you can see clearly, usually within a day, but sometimes it takes a few days to a week.

- Sunglasses should be worn for the first few days or until bright light no longer is a bother.

- You can read and watch TV, but do so in moderation.

- Do not wear eye makeup for the first week. You don't want to risk having flecks of mascara or eye shadow floating in your eye.

- Avoid swimming pools, hot tubs, and whirlpools for the first week.

- Avoid gardening and dusty environments for the first week.

- For several weeks avoid contact sports such as football, basketball, rugby, or any activity that could result in injury to the eye.

- Smoking is okay, but your eyes probably will be sensitive to the smoke for a while.

Common sense should rule. If you are not comfortable while engaged in some activity, stop. Over the next few weeks you will notice a dramatic change in your vision; enjoy. The gift of sight is a wonder.

7

Is Laser Vision Correction Safe?

It's increasingly common to hear about or meet someone who has had laser vision correction. Most former patients enthusiastically endorse the procedure and without encouragement will tell anyone who will listen that it's one of the best things they've ever done for themselves. This often is true even when patients experienced complications during surgery, when it took longer than expected for their vision to stabilize, or when a second procedure was required to achieve the very best possible results.

There also are patients who are not happy with their results, people with significant complications, or at least the people considered them significant, and whose resulting visual problems are persistent. These stories tend to travel quickly, and the patient's problem grows in severity with each retelling of the tale. As the story gets told and retold, the ability and intention of the treating surgeon come under suspicion. Anyone who searches the Internet can find stories of "greedy," "incompetent" ophthalmologists permanently ruining a patient's vision, all for the accumulation of a few more dollars, or so is the conclusion drawn by those who retell these tales.

Although doctors, like all of us who work for a living, certainly gain satisfaction from being well compensated for their education, training, and expertise, very few would perform an elective surgical procedure on someone just for the money, regardless of its safety or effectiveness.

No eye doctor who wished to continue practicing would recommend an elective procedure, for which most patients pay out of pocket, if he or she wasn't confident in its safety and effectiveness.

When a physician enters the profession, he or she promises to "first, do no harm." It's called the Hippocratic Oath and is an ethical obligation to do what is in the best interest of the patient. Doctors take that charge very seriously.

No responsible doctor would encourage any patient to undergo a procedure of questionable safety unless the alternative was worse, such as certain death. And certainly no eye doctor who wished to continue practicing would recommend an elective procedure, for which most patients pay out of pocket, if he or she wasn't confident in its safety and effectiveness.

Dr. Brint says most emphatically that "I frequently dissuade patients who think they are good candidates from having the procedure if it's really not right for them. I also discourage prospective patients if they don't really understand the ramifications of their decision, such as maybe needing reading glasses for near vision when they didn't before because they were able to use their nearsightedness to read without glasses. Treating the wrong patient can only come back to haunt you."

We've said it before, but it can't be said too often. Treating patients who should not be treated isn't good medicine, and it isn't good business.

Pioneers Push the Envelope

Of course, there are doctors who pioneer new areas of medicine, such as those who developed and refined refractive surgery techniques over the past 100 years. And there are physicians today in all areas of medicine who "push the envelope" of current practice by experimenting with product use or surgical techniques, but they do so from a firm foundation of knowledge and experience. Sometimes these unproven techniques are less successful than anticipated; sometimes they are more successful than the doctor's wildest imagination. That's how medical breakthroughs are accomplished. And that's why one day every person who so chooses will be able to have any refractive error surgically corrected.

Because some surgeons are willing to take some risks and freely share the results with their colleagues, treatment parameters are expanded for all patients. For example, Dr. Brint traveled the globe observing other refractive surgeons performing LASIK and attending conferences where the results of others' efforts were shared. In 1991 he became the first refractive surgeon in the United States to perform LASIK on a sighted eye during a clinical investigation. This was four years before the FDA approved the excimer laser for use in PRK. (See chapter 10 for a discussion of clinical investigations.) Since then he has taught hundreds of other surgeons, lectured to thousands of doctors around the world, and written two textbooks with Lucio Barrato, M.D., a refractive surgeon practicing in Italy who in 1990 was the first in the world to perform LASIK.

Discovery is just that, and it happens because experienced doctors are willing to take small risks to build a foundation for common practice. Among the early patients treated with the excimer laser in the United States by Dr. Marguerite McDonald was a women who was blind in one eye; the FDA required that the first eyes treated in the clinical trials be blind. Only, as it turns out, she wasn't. The blindness was psychological, not physiological. It was a rare case of hysterical blindness.

That she was not blind was discovered when Dr. McDonald performed PRK on the blind eye during clinical trials of the VISX laser. Because she believed the women to be blind in the treated eye, and she was eager to learn the effect of the laser on corneal tissue when programmed for a full correction, Dr. McDonald programmed into the laser's computer the correction to be achieved if the eye were sighted. She used the woman's last known prescription as the target correction. Days after the surgery, the woman called to tell the doctor the astonishing news that not only could she see out of the treated eye, she could see clearly. Dr. McDonald was willing to push the envelope just a little to take a giant leap forward in current knowledge. Taking risks and learning from the results often are in the best interests of not just the patient being treated but of all future patients with similar conditions.

Fortunately, the vast majority of patients treated for refractive error need routine care. And for the small minority who require special attention, the alternative, which is to forgo surgery and continue using corrective lenses, is considered by them to be the greater of the two challenges.

Regulatory Protection

To some degree, patients are protected from harm by the regulatory requirements imposed on manufacturers of medical products and devices by the U.S. Food and Drug Administration (FDA). Before any medical device or product can be sold commercially in the United States, its manufacturer must prove to the satisfaction of the FDA that it is safe and effective. The agency is guided in its decision by advisory panels composed of physicians who specialize in the area of medicine in which the product or device ultimately will be used. (See chapter 10 for a complete discussion of the FDA approval process.)

Approval for products and devices to be used in cosmetic or elective surgery, or for what are called "lifestyle" drugs such as those used for obesity and hair loss, are held to a much higher safety standard than are products or devices used to treat life-threatening or life-compromising conditions. This is because use of such devices and products is discretionary and because the opportunity for misuse of products designed for elective or cosmetic treatments is believed to be greater than it is for other products.

Doctors Choose Laser Vision Correction

It's true—no one has to have refractive surgery. Contact lenses and eyeglasses are usually adequate to correct the conditions for which they are prescribed. This is why laser vision correction is considered a cosmetic procedure. However, as anyone with poor vision can tell you, depending on corrective lenses can be a life-threatening handicap. More often it is inconvenient, uncomfortable, unsatisfying, and restrictive. And many people who wear corrective lenses insist that as a result they feel less attractive and less confident. That's why they elect to have refractive surgery, and that's why many eye doctors recommend laser vision correction.

That's also why doctors in every area of medicine have their own eyes treated with the excimer laser, as did my co-author, Steve Brint, M.D. And maybe this is the best measure of just how safe and effective it is as a treatment for refractive error: Doctors are choosing to have laser vision correction. It should be particularly reassuring that so many ophthalmologists and optometrists are having laser vision correction, considering that their careers are devoted to the diagnosis and treatment of vision problems. Furthermore, ophthalmic surgeons must have exceptionally good vision because they perform surgery under a microscope on a surface area that is measured in millimeters. They also treat or refer their families, coworkers, and friends.

> *It should be particularly reassuring that so many ophthalmologists and optometrists are having laser vision correction, considering that their careers are devoted to the diagnosis and treatment of vision problems.*

Comments Dr. Brint, "Studies show that the more doctors, especially eye doctors, know about laser vision correction, the more likely they are to have it performed on themselves. Some 40 percent of high-volume refractive surgeons who once depended on corrective lenses have had refractive surgery after seeing the great results they achieved for their patients day in and day out. That's why I chose it for myself."

In your own research into laser vision correction, you may have come across some of the Internet sites that paint a very negative picture of refractive surgery and refractive surgeons. One such sight, eyeknowwhy.com, which is shorthand for "I know why doctors wear eyeglasses," relentlessly hammers home the point that while many ophthalmologists and optometrists are happy to recommend refractive surgery to their patients, they aren't willing to "go under the knife" themselves. That may have been true when radial keratotomy (RK) was the predominant surgical option for low and moderate refractive errors, but it certainly is no longer true. Thousands of doctors in every branch of medicine have elected to have their vision corrected with PRK or LASIK.

Among TLC's network of 11,000 eye doctors, 1,000 have had their vision corrected with the laser, and 2,000 doctors in other areas of medicine also have come to TLC centers to have their vision corrected. Countless others recommend the procedure to spouses, children, siblings, and parents.

Perception Versus Reality

Most providers of laser vision correction take great pains to educate potential patients about the procedure. This includes an in-depth discussion of likely symptoms post-surgery and the risks associated with refractive procedures, to ensure that patients are fully prepared for what will happen and what could happen. This is a critical component of good patient care. The alternative is unhappy patients who may see as well as, or even better than, they did before refractive surgery, but because they were unprepared, they now perceive themselves to be worse off.

Many doctors tell stories of patients with postsurgery visual acuity of 20/20 without glasses or contact lenses, and no clinical evidence of a vision problem, who are certain their vision is worse than when it was corrected to 20/20 with lenses. They complain of symptoms such as blurring, glare, or vision fluctuations as if they never experienced any of these when wearing corrective lenses, although they probably did. For them, perception becomes reality.

I have spoken with patients who had a complication during or after surgery who told me with great passion that no one explained to them that these things could happen. When asked about the informed consent, all confirm that they read and signed the document but were led to believe that the likelihood of any one of those problems occurring was so remote as to be not worthy of discussion.

Certainly, sometimes patients didn't pay attention or chose to believe that certain complications couldn't possibly happen to them! Dr. Machat asserts that people who truly believe that they might have a complication ultimately decide not to have the procedure. He thinks that it's human nature to believe that bad things won't happen and that anyone who really thinks something bad will happen makes a different choice than someone who is convinced that nothing bad will happen. But more often, it is the case that the doctor or the doctor's staff downplayed the risks for fear of scaring away a patient, which is not a good idea.

Fortunately, for most patients surgery is anxiety producing but otherwise uneventful. The vast majority of people recover quickly; experience very few, if any, postoperative symptoms; and go on to enjoy corrective lens–free vision. However, virtually every patient is in a heightened state of awareness before and, particularly, just after surgery. If the patient is not properly prepared for the symptoms commonly experienced postsurgery or is not educated about symptoms suggesting serious complications, then every minor fluctuation in vision and every perceived aberration becomes a cause for concern.

If you are like most patients, within a few hours of the procedure, you will begin "testing" your visual acuity. First, you will challenge yourself to see things you never could see before without corrective lenses, such as fine print scrolling across the television screen or book titles on shelves across the room. Next, you will test each eye separately, covering first one eye, then the other. Inevitably, you will determine that one eye is healing "better or faster" than is the other. It probably isn't. Some patients will then conclude that something is wrong with the eye that they determine to be not responding as quickly. There probably isn't.

The fact is that every single person experiences laser vision correction differently, and every single patient heals differently. Says Dr. Machat, "How the patient will respond is the Achilles' heel of refractive surgery. It is what prevents doctors from achieving the exact same results with the exact same nomograms on two patients with the exact same prescription. So, the best we can do is prepare the patient for all possibilities, knowing that most of them will emerge with excellent vision."

Optometrist Harry Snyder suggests that people contemplating refractive surgery might want to try on their own, or with their doctor's cooperation, the following visual test before they have surgery:

Take your eyeglasses off and really pay attention to what you can and can't see and from what distance. Try to read fine print on the television screen or computer monitor without them. See which book titles you can or can't read from across the room. Test first one eye and then the other, and see if vision in one eye is clearer than the other. You probably will find that one is better than the other and that it might not always be the same one.

Also, try to notice how your vision changes from the time you get up in the morning until the time you go to sleep at night. Note the environmental factors that contribute to a change in vision, such as dim light, the dark of night, or weather conditions. Note how your work habits affect your vision, such as staring at a computer screen for long periods of time. If you make yourself more keenly aware of your vision prior to surgery, you will be less unsettled when your vision isn't perfect just after. And it won't be. Right after the procedure, it will be as if someone has smeared Vaseline over your eyeglass lenses. With each passing hour, a bit more of the Vaseline will be wiped away until you are able to see clearly without corrective lenses.

The Good, the Bad, and the Ugly

But getting back to the original question, Is laser vision correction safe? The short answer is yes, it is safe and effective, and the results are reasonably predictable, but as is true of any surgery, patients who have refractive surgery are at risk of experiencing one or several complications. Most of these are mild but on occasion can be severe. Patients are very likely to experience some common surgical side effects or postoperative symptoms. Virtually all of them can be managed, sometimes by the patient, more often under the supervision of the doctor providing postoperative care.

> *The short answer is yes, it is safe and effective, and the results are reasonably predictable, but as is true of any surgery, patients who have refractive surgery are at risk of experiencing one or several complications.*

When lecturing to other doctors about refractive surgery and when speaking with potential patients, Dr. Roy Rubinfeld divides surgical and postoperative symptoms and complications into three categories:

- The good—normal healing reactions, including glare, sensitivity to light, and undercorrection or overcorrection
- The bad—significant complications that need to be treated
- The ugly—serious, usually preventable, complications that occur as a result of inexperience, laziness, and inattention to detail or poor judgment on the part of the surgeon

Most problems fall into one of the first two categories. For example, most patients experience, to a lesser or greater degree, mild discomfort, which is sometimes referred to as a foreign-body sensation. Most also experience dry eyes, sensitivity to light (photophobia), and blurred and/or fluctuating vision. These symptoms almost always resolve themselves quickly unless there is some other problem, which we will get to shortly.

PRK patients might be uncomfortable for twenty-four to forty-eight hours, LASIK patients for four to twenty-four hours. Many LASIK and some PRK patients experience no discomfort at all. However, if they do, usually an over-the-counter pain medication such as Tylenol or Advil eases the symptoms. Also, a cold compress on your closed eyelids can soothe that scratchy feeling, particularly if you also rest in a dark room.

Light sensitivity is managed by wearing wraparound sunglasses and by staying away from bright lights, at least for the first day or so. Dry eyes can be soothed with artificial tears, and blurred or fluctuating vision eases in time. Some patients see clearly on day one; others take a week or more to achieve visual clarity. And even then, vision might still fluctuate for a few months, with changes most often noticed in the early morning hours and in the evening.

Longer-lasting side effects, such as glare and halos around bright lights at night, also are quite common and usually resolve themselves without medical intervention. Glare, starbursts, or halos are a result of irregularities in the cornea or pupils that, when fully dilated, are larger than the area treated, the optical zone. If a patient has unusually large dilated pupils, larger than the treatment zone, then light will fragment at the perimeter where the ablated area meets untouched corneal tissue. For these patients glare is persistent and can cause significant problems, particularly making night driving a challenge.

Some of these patients can be helped by traveling to a center that has a "flying spot" laser. Autonomous Technologies and LaserSight Technologies both manufacture "flying spot" lasers that have been approved by the FDA for use in PRK, although neither are in as widespread use as the lasers manufactured by VISX and Summit Technologies. "Flying spot" lasers can be programmed to treat a wider optical zone, up to 10 millimeters, which might correct the problem. (See chapter 9 for a discussion of developing technology.)

If you know people who have this problem and who have cautioned you against having laser vision correction because of it, you may want to tell them to ask their doctor or the center where they were treated whether they can be referred to a trial site or to another center.

Most of the time, glare and halos are corneal flap–related, because most refractive surgeons are careful not to treat patients with extremely large pupils.

Although the flap begins to adhere to the cornea immediately after surgery and can only be dislodged with some effort, such as through a trauma to the eye, it can take a week or so for the flap to "settle" into place. Until it does, there can be irregularities on the cornea. Think of them like minuscule wrinkles or bubbles; when bright light hits these irregularities, it fragments and creates a starburst effect.

Sometimes irregularities persist. This is called an irregular astigmatism, which causes light to enter the eye at two or more points. Some people have naturally occurring irregular astigmatism, but more often people have astigmatism that results from a cornea that is oval-shaped like a football, rather than round like a baseball. (See chapter 3 for a more complete discussion of astigmatism.)

Again, most of the time, irregular astigmatism disappears without treatment over a period of weeks or months. Rarely, it persists and causes a permanent loss of best corrected visual acuity (BCVA). (See chapter 6 for an explanation of BCVA.) To achieve the very best vision possible, the corneal surface has to be smooth. When an irregular astigmatism is present, the cornea is not smooth. Furthermore, eyeglasses and soft contact lenses cannot correct for irregular astigmatism. Rigid gas-permeable contact lenses can, but for people who could not wear contact lenses prior to surgery, that would not be an option.

Enhancements

Dr. Rubinfeld includes undercorrection or overcorrection in the "good" category, because both are easily remedied with a second procedure. Surgeons make every effort to achieve the desired correction on the first attempt; however, that is not always possible. It is particularly difficult for patients with higher degrees of refractive error.

Referred to variously as retreatment, enhancement, touch-up, or tweaking, second procedures are necessary for 10 to 20 percent of patients and are more common in patients with higher degrees of refractive errors. Experienced, high-volume surgeons tend to have lower enhancement rates than do inexperienced surgeons. This is because they have learned over time how to adjust targeted correction based on a patient's age, known health conditions that might affect the healing response, and desired outcome based on a patient's lifestyle and the environment of the room in which the laser is housed. Lasers behave differently in various climates and altitudes, especially in cities as different as Miami, Florida, and Denver, Colorado.

As Dr. Whitten explains: "The number of laser pulses required to achieve a specific correction is different in Denver than it is in Miami because of the altitude and the humidity of the general atmosphere. When you work on a laser in a room in which you control the atmosphere to some degree, you learn how the laser behaves in that particular environment. The surgeon adjusts his or her nomograms—the formula to achieve desired correction—accordingly.

"A surgeon's nomograms usually reduce the amount of correction that is programmed into the laser by anywhere from 10 to 20 percent. It's important to note that the amount of the reduction doesn't really matter that much in patients with up to about 6.00 diopters of correction near- or far-sighted, because 10 to 20 percent of 6.00 diopters is a small amount. However, when you get up to 15.00, then you are talking about 1.00 to 2.00 diopters' difference, depending on whether you change your nomogram by 10, 20, or 30 percent, which depends on the patient's level of correction. Everything matters more the more nearsighted or farsighted you are. And that's the real challenge.

"Age makes a difference in deciding whether to err on the conservative or the more aggressive side—whether you want to err on the nearsighted side or the farsighted side. If you are treating a younger patient, you can afford to aim closer. You can afford to make a nearsighted person far-sighted because he or she will be able to focus through it. When the patient is older, you can't afford to do that so you have to err more on the nearsighted side. That's why when you are dealing with a patient who is over 45, you take a look at the formulas that you have and if you have any question, you're always going to reduce the amount that you correct in a nearsighted person. If anything, you err on the nearsighted side. Then if you have to retreat the person, you know that you won't overcorrect. You know that your nomogram will be within one-tenth of a diopter or two-tenths of a diopter, the 20-percent range."

In the early days, when the excimer laser was first approved for use in PRK, retreatment rates were much higher than they are today. All surgeons erred on the more conservative, or nearsighted, side because the laser was not approved for use in the treatment of hyperopia, or farsight-edness. If a patient was overcorrected, there were not too many options available. Some surgeons in Canada used what is known as a holmium laser to treat overcorrection, but the results were not always satisfactory. (See chapter 9 for a more complete description of the holmium laser.) It was far better to undercorrect and retreat than to end up with an unhappy, farsighted patient.

Potentially Serious Complications

Then there are the unwanted incidents, what Dr. Rubinfeld calls the "bad" complications that occur during surgery or as a result of the patient's healing response. In PRK, serious complications are more likely to occur during the healing process than during surgery. In LASIK, serious complications are more likely to occur intraoperatively (during surgery).

In PRK, serious complications are more likely to occur during the healing process than during surgery.

The least common, but potentially most dangerous, complication associated with PRK and LASIK is infection. Because antibiotic eyedrops are administered routinely as a preventive measure, the incidence of infection is extremely rare. In fact, serious vision-compromising infections are far more common among contact lens wearers than among refractive surgery patients.

Statistics vary slightly by source, but the incidence of corneal infection among contact lens wearers is about 1 in 500 for those with extended wear lenses, and 1 in 2,500 for wearers of daily soft contacts and rigid gas-permeable lenses. Among those who wear daily non–gas permeable hard contact lenses, the incidence of infection is about 1 in 5,000. According to the LASIK Institute, a study of 1,062 eyes conducted by ophthalmologists at Emory University revealed complications in 2.6 percent of all procedures post-operatively, with not a single incidence of infection.

Both PRK and LASIK patients are at very small risk for what is called a decentered ablation, which means that the area of the cornea from which tissue is removed during laser treatment surgery is not aligned with the patient's pupil. When this happens, some of the light that enters the eye will be focused and some will not be. This can cause patients to lose visual acuity and quality of vision, some-times reducing their contrast sensitivity, making vision less sharp. Decentered ablations, which are extremely rare, occur when the laser beam is not properly centered on the pupil during the procedure. Sometimes it is because the patient moved, and sometimes it is because the surgeon is inexperienced. "Even more rarely," adds Dr. Brint, "it is because the laser optics are not properly aligned."

During PRK and LASIK, it is critical that you follow the surgeon's instructions to stare at the blinking red, or green, light, depending on which laser is in use. Slight movements won't affect outcome, but significant movement might. However, don't become overly anxious about this. The surgeon is in complete control of the laser at all times. If you move and the surgeon believes that the outcome will be affected, he or she will stop the procedure, realign the laser beam, and instruct you to stare at the light. The laser's computer will remember exactly where the procedure was halted and will resume from that point.

Probably the most serious complications associated with PRK are haze and irregular astigmatism, discussed previously; the latter can be a result of abnormal healing of the corneal surface. Earlier lasers produced central islands in some patients, which were areas of the cornea that did not receive the full impact of the laser beam, usually centrally right over the pupil, and so were not fully corrected. However, technological improvements in the laser have greatly reduced the incidence of central islands. Such uneven removal of corneal tissue has not been as much of a problem with LASIK.

Haze is detectable under the high-powered microscope of the slit lamp. It gives the cornea a milky or grainy appearance but isn't usually noticed by the patient unless it is significant. If it is, it can result in blurred vision and reduced quality of vision. Haze is graded, with minimal or trace amounts graded as 0.0 to 0.5; mild haze as 1.0 to 1.5; moderate as 2.0; and severe as 3.0. Treatment for haze ranges from no treatment at all to increased use of eyedrops called corticosteroids, with such names as Flarex and Inflamase Forte. PRK patients are routinely given these drops for anywhere from a few weeks to a few months, to control postoperative inflammation. LASIK patients generally use these drops for only a few days.

If haze persists, doctors generally prescribe increased use of topical steroids over a longer period of time. Although haze can rarely occur in LASIK patients, it is more commonly associated with PRK.

Flap Complications

In LASIK, most complications occur during the creation of the flap of corneal tissue or are flap-related. As described in the previous chapter, one possible flap-related complication is the creation of a "free cap," which means there is no hinge of tissue, and the flap becomes detached from the eye. Newer microkeratomes are designed to minimize free caps; however, there are still lots of older units in use that may have a slightly higher incidence of free caps.

Other complications that might occur during the creation of the flap include incomplete flaps, which means the flap is too small and if folded over would not leave sufficient room for the excimer ablation; flaps that are too thin; and perforated (buttonhole) or torn caps. Sometimes the corneal tissue becomes tangled in the microkeratome as it passes backward over the cornea. When this happens, the surgeon recovers the pieces of tissue and places the tissue back over the stroma. The procedure is stopped and the patient is sent home. In most cases, the patient can be treated at a later date.

An experienced surgeon can easily manage each of these flap complications. For example, if a "free cap" is intact and of sufficient thickness, the surgeon is likely to complete the ablation (removal of the corneal tissue with the excimer laser), put the flap back in place over the stroma, and send the patient home to heal. And remember from the last chapter, the cornea is marked with a water-soluble ink to ensure that the cap is properly positioned after surgery. If a cap becomes free, the surgeon is able to replace the cap by lining up the marks.

Dr. Brint reminds us that "This is the way it was routinely done for years before the concept of the hinge emerged; thus, to an experienced surgeon, a free cap is a nuisance rather than a complication." Any other flap complication probably means that the surgeon will discontinue the procedure for that day, repair the damaged tissue, and send the patient home. Once the cornea has had a chance to heal, the patient can again undergo the procedure. Most surgeons wait about three months before making a second attempt. Flap complications occur in 1 to 2 percent of patients.

When you are interviewing doctors or their staff during the selection process, an important question to ask is "What percentage of your patients experience flap-related complications during surgery?" If the answer is none, walk away. Every single surgeon occasionally creates a poor flap for any number of reasons, including equipment failure, inadequate pressure during the microkeratome pass, jostling of the instrument when it is in use, or because of a defective blade. These things do happen. Quoting Dr. Machat again: "If doctors say they have never had a complication, they either don't do surgery or they are lying."

Postsurgery LASIK Complications

Immediately after surgery or within the first twenty-four hours, it is possible for the corneal flap to become dislocated or, even more rarely, lost. When it does, it is usually a result of trauma to the eye or because, while sleeping, the patient rubbed his or her eyes. One patient lost a corneal flap when his young son took a tumble and elbowed him in the eye just after surgery.

If the corneal flap becomes dislodged, you'll know it because you will feel extreme pain and your vision will be very blurry. This complication must be treated at once. If it happens after normal business hours, call the emergency number supplied by your doctor or the laser center. If you are unable to reach someone there, go to the emergency room and tell the desk attendant that you just had refractive surgery and you need to be seen by an ophthalmologist experienced in refractive surgery.

Most of the time, dislodged or dislocated flaps can be repositioned with no long-term vision problems resulting. Lost caps may have to be replaced with donor corneal tissue or may be allowed to heal similar to a PRK. For an ophthalmic surgeon this is a fairly routine surgical procedure, and, unlike human organs, donor corneal tissue is not difficult to come by.

Other post-LASIK complications happen during the healing process. Some can be quite serious if not treated quickly and appropriately, even leading to blindness.

Again, let us reassure you that there are no reported cases of permanent blindness resulting from PRK or LASIK surgical or postsurgical complications. A few people have experienced complications serious enough to require a corneal transplant to restore vision. And there have been instances of a reduction in BCVA of one or two lines, as well as persistent glare, double vision, loss of contrast sensitivity, and irregular astigmatism. These incidents account for less than 1 percent of the millions of patients who have had their vision corrected with the excimer laser.

However, complications from refractive surgery can become extremely serious if left untreated. This is why it is extremely important that you keep all of your follow-up appointments even if your vision seems fine.

Flap Folds and Epithelial Ingrowth

One of the things your doctor looks for during your first postoperative visit, usually within twenty-four hours of your procedure, are folds in the corneal flap. These are called wrinkles or striae. They can result from the cap being improperly positioned just after surgery or from the cap being dislocated by rubbing or hitting the eye. If folds are present during your post-op visit, your doctor will reposition the flap and the problem will be solved. The longer a fold remains, the harder it is to resolve the problem. Although doctors have successfully repositioned wrinkled flaps months after surgery, this can result in irregular astigmatism. Of course, it's better to catch the problem earlier rather than later.

It also is possible for epithelial cells to grow underneath the corneal flap. As you probably remember from an earlier chapter, the epithelium is the top layer of corneal tissue. It is four to five cell layers thick. After being wounded in refractive surgery, either by being removed as it is during PRK or lifted as part of the flap, the epithelium regenerates itself. In rare cases, epithelial cells grow under rather than over the corneal flap. This is called epithelial ingrowth.

When this occurs, the surgeon will lift the flap, wipe away the cells, and reposition the flap. Usually, healing continues with no further complications and the patient's vision is not affected. If left untreated, however, the result can be distorted vision from pronounced irregular astigmatism and a permanent loss of BCVA. This problem occurs more often in patients with loose epithelium that is easily dislodged. The risk of epithelial ingrowth also is higher with enhancements when the existing flap is lifted rather than a new flap being cut because the surgeon must lift the already created flap and reposition it, disturbing the newly regenerated epithelial cells.

In addition to the risk of epithelial cells growing under the flap, there also is a risk that tiny fragments, or debris, will be trapped under the flap during surgery. Most of the time when this occurs, the patient is completely unaware, although the doctor can see the debris through the slit lamp, and it has no impact on visual outcome. When there is cause for concern, the surgeon will lift the flap, remove the debris, and reposition the flap, taking great care that the flap realigns properly.

A very rare, but potentially serious, complication is known as diffuse interface keratitis, also called Sands of the Sahara, which is an accumulation of cells that gives the cornea a cloudy appearance that looks like swirling, shifting sand. Doctors are unsure what exactly causes this problem, but it is believed to be an immune or toxic reaction. It is treated with steroid eyedrops. If it persists, the surgeon will lift the flap, clean out the interface, and put the flap back in place. Untreated, it can cause serious, vision-compromising problems including, in the extreme, the need for a corneal transplant or blindness.

The Ugly—Usually Preventable Problems

Dr. Rubinfeld refers to preventable LASIK complications as "ugly," mostly because they occur as a result of insufficient attention to detail. He includes among these: failing to attach and secure the microkeratome plate; performing a procedure when the plate is not properly positioned; applying the laser when there is an incomplete, thin, irregular, or button-holed flap; or excessive time under suction, which creates other ocular problems.

There have been one or two cases in which surgeons failed to ensure that the microkeratome depth plate was in the instrument prior to use. As a result the cornea was perforated. Even this is treatable, although recovery can take many months. Using a defective blade in the microkeratome also can create serious problems, with torn caps and irregular astigmatism the most common result.

Incidents of such ugly complications are extremely rare. Most surgeons and most laser centers treat every single patient and every procedure as if it were the only one to be done that day. Surgeons and technicians check the refractive numbers to be programmed into the laser at many different points in the process. And each monitors the other as a safety mechanism and a double-check. After a technician has checked the microkeratome blade for defects, the surgeon often checks again. A technician will assemble the microkeratome; the surgeon checks to make sure it is properly assembled, that proper suction can be maintained, and that the gears move freely. These steps are repeated between the two procedures in a bilateral operation and between patients.

Other Complications

If you haven't read enough already, there are a few other potential complications that should be mentioned. Some patients develop a droopy upper eyelid after LASIK surgery. This is called ptosis and is caused when the eyelid speculum used to hold your lids open during the procedure stretches the muscle responsible for opening the eyelid. When stretched, the muscle sometimes becomes irritated, causing the eyelid to droop and the eye to appear smaller. Usually, this goes away in just a few days. If it persists, however, it can be corrected with eyelid surgery.

> *Other post-LASIK complications happen during the healing process. Some can be quite serious if not treated quickly and appropriately, even leading to blindness.*

It is possible for patients to experience a temporary increase in intraocular pressure, which is one of the reasons why people who have uncontrolled glaucoma are not good candidates for the procedure. Glaucoma is a condition in which the pressure inside the eye is elevated. Long-term, this can result in damage to the optic nerve and loss of vision. This problem most frequently occurs in people found to be "steroid responders," which means that the eyedrops they take to control inflammation after surgery cause the increase in pressure. Treatment often is nothing more than a discontinuation of the eyedrops.

Some patients who choose to have only one eye treated experience a condition called anisometropia, which means that their two eyes together don't focus in the same place. Some also experience aniseikonia, which is a difference in the size of images created by the two eyes. Both can cause symptoms such as nausea, eyestrain, headache, double vision, and difficulty with depth perception. Unless patients then decide to have the other eye treated, they will normally have to wear a contact lens or, less commonly, eyeglasses, which don't work very well to correct this problem.

Increased risk for cataracts is sometimes said to be a complication of LASIK, but there is no data to support this. In any case, a direct correlation between refractive surgery and cataracts would be difficult to prove, as many people develop cataracts later in life and it would be hard to assess which patients would have developed them even if they had never had laser vision correction.

Finally, some patients will find that their refractive correction regresses over time. Although, laser vision correction permanently corrects refractive errors; it cannot stop the aging process. Some people become increasingly myopic or hyperopic as they age. The laser can't change your physiological predisposition. In other words, if you were going to become more myopic or hyperopic over time, you most likely will after refractive surgery. If the change becomes significant enough, you can have another laser procedure to correct the resulting refractive error as long as there is no other medical problem that would prevent you from having surgery.

> *Although, laser vision correction permanently corrects refractive errors; it cannot stop the aging process.*

Frequency of Complications

Now that you know everything that could go wrong during and after surgery, my co-authors and I want to reassure you that the incidence of complications is exceedingly low. In clinical trials prior to FDA approval of the excimer laser for use in PRK, VISX, and Summit, patients experienced complication rates of less than 1 percent for all serious, sight-compromising problems.

In its discussion of risks and complications, the LASIK Institute reports on the results of three studies, revealing the following:

As of April 1, 1998, the CRS-USA LASIK study that considered 1,800 eyes noted two complications that arose during the procedures themselves resulting from the microkeratome: irregular cuts damaging the stromal bed (experienced by 0.03% of the patient population) and damage to the epithelium (0.47%). Two complications required patients to forgo treatment or return another day but did not cause loss of visual acuity: flaps were too small (0.38%) or too thin (0.38%). All of the aforementioned complications produced temporary effects. After 3 months, the visual results of the group experiencing intra-operative complications were no different from the group who experienced no such complications.

In January, 1999, the results of the Emory Study that considered 1,062 eyes and 1,530 surgical procedures were published. The study noted a 1.8% intra-operative complication rate. Seventeen eyes had to postpone treatment that day due to flap complications. Only 3 eyes lost 2 or more Snellen lines of best corrected visual acuity.

A study conducted by Doctors Lin and Maloney that considered 1,019 eyes for which a flap was created by means of a microkeratome noted a 2.2% intra-operative complication rate. However, no eyes suffered permanent decrease in visual acuity because of flap complications.

The CRS-USA LASIK Study noted that overall, 5.8% of LASIK patients experienced complications at the three-month follow-up period that did not result from complications during the procedure itself. These complications included corneal edema [swelling] (0.6%), corneal scarring (0.1%), persistent epithelial defect (0.5%), significant glare (0.2%), persistent discomfort or pain (0.5%), interface epithelium (0.6%), cap thinning (0.1%), and interface debris (3.2%). It is important to note that interface debris—retained metallic particles, lint, etc., under the flap—almost always causes no harm to the health or vision of the eye. None of these complications resulted in a loss of two or more lines of BCVA, and there was no incidence of infection amongst the study population.

The Emory Study, on the other hand, observed complications in only 2.6 percent of all procedures postoperatively. Only one eye lost two or more lines of BCVA, and this eye had postoperative flap folds. There was no evidence of infection in any of the patients treated.

In others words, complications do happen, but they are infrequent and when they do occur, experienced doctors are able to manage the problem with no long-lasting impact on vision.

So, what can you expect? According to Dr. Machat, "What patients need to know is that the most common symptom postsurgery is dry eyes, the most common side effect is glare, and the most common complication resulting from a patient's healing response is irregularities of the cornea that cause a reduction in visual clarity. And the most common flap complication during surgery is a button-hole flap, which is caused by insufficient suction."

When asked if there were data charts that displayed the risk of each side effect, symptom, or complication at different degrees of refractive errors, Dr. Machat answered that "because every single patient heals differently, it is not possible to create such a chart. A good, very general rule of thumb is the higher the degree of refractive error, the more time under the laser, the greater the likelihood that the patient will experience a problem. But no one can say for sure which patient will have a problem and which patient won't. What we do know is that the more experienced a surgeon is, the less likely there will be a problem. And when a problem does occur, experienced doctors know how to manage it to avoid permanent loss of vision."

8

What Can I Expect to Pay for Laser Vision Correction?

Procedure costs vary significantly from region to region and from provider to provider. In many ways laser vision correction is very much a local business, and costs can depend on how many providers are competing for the same procedure dollars.

Some patients have paid as little as $500 for each eye; others have paid $3,000 or more. At least one surgeon in the Philadelphia, Pennsylvania, area bases his fee on the patient's level of needed correction. He charges a lower fee for the treatment of low to moderate refractive errors and a higher fee for higher degrees of refractive error.

Dr. Brint notes that "The reason for charging higher fees for higher degrees of refractive error probably is based on the fact that touch-ups or enhancements are much more common in high corrections than in low corrections (20 percent versus almost none). The cost to the surgeon for an enhancement is the same as the cost associated with the original procedure. The only cost that is not a factor the second time around is the Pillar Point royalty fee. Neither VISX nor Summit collects the $250 Pillar Point fee for a second procedure on the same eye. The other costs, such as technician salaries, laser gases, microkeratome blades, and other disposable items, are the same."

The Pillar Point fee is paid to an entity known as the Pillar Point Partnership, which was established by VISX and Summit Technology as a means of ensuring that neither would sue the other for patent infringement over the development of two very similar excimer lasers. The partnership and the $250-per-use royalty fee are extremely controversial and the focus of innumerable lawsuits filed by other manufacturers, by physicians, and by some consumer advocacy groups.

Why Fees Vary

Facilities owned by management companies such as TLC Laser Eye Centers tend to have standardized fees, with perhaps some slight regional variations. Often surgeons will sign a contract with the management company under which they agree to pay a fixed fee for each use of the laser. That fee covers administrative support services, technician support, materials, equipment, and other costs associated with managing a health-care facility.

The total fee paid by a patient at the time of the procedure, also called a global fee, includes that facility fee, as well as fees for professional services rendered by the surgeon and the co–managing doctor.

Generally speaking, fees paid for procedures performed at one of these laser centers is higher for LASIK than for PRK, and higher still for hyperopic and sometimes for astigmatic treatment.

Teaching hospitals often charge less than do management companies or private-practice physicians because they can afford to. Many hospital administrators view excimer lasers as they do any new technology: essential equipment they must have to be perceived as competitive.

However, they don't necessarily view the business of refractive surgery as a profit center the way they might cardiac care or cancer treatments. They may also use the laser as a "loss leader" to attract surgeons to use their facility for other eye operations such as cataracts.

> *The total fee paid by a patient at the time of the procedure, also called a global fee, includes that facility fee, as well as fees for professional services rendered by the surgeon and the co–managing doctor.*

Generating sufficient patient volume to realize a return on the investment in an excimer laser, which costs around $500,000, plus another $75,000 to $100,000 annually in supplies such as gas and maintenance, takes more marketing savvy and dollars than most teaching hospitals care to spend. To earn back that investment, a hospital would have to generate enough patients for the laser to pay for itself. That takes marketing dollars, which, once spent, also have to be earned back.

Consequently, many hospitals, particularly teaching hospitals, make the laser available to staff ophthalmic surgeons for a fee and also use it to teach residents, but they don't necessarily concern themselves with building a reputation as laser vision correction specialists. With the profit motive minimized, procedure costs can be reduced. Surgeons then are free to charge whatever fee they determine to be appropriate—truthfully, whatever the market will bear.

Independent surgeons and group practices with in-office lasers often compete on price, hoping to recover revenues once they build reputations as refractive surgeons.

In densely populated areas where there are facilities owned by one or more national management company chains, as well as physician-owned lasers and hospitals with lasers, it is very likely that there will be dramatic price differences and that costs will fluctuate in response to the pricing strategies of others.

In these regions, mostly large metropolitan areas such as Washington, D.C.; New York; Chicago; Los Angeles; and Miami, it is fairly common to receive direct-mail solicitations or come across newspaper advertisements offering what amounts to a dollars-off coupon. Many times, the dollars-off inducement is presented as a special lower professional fee for patients willing to participate in a study. Very likely, the doctor is involved in an ongoing study of some sort. Many doctors participate in studies for pharmaceutical companies, laser manufacturers, or makers of other ophthalmic devices. There isn't anything wrong with the strategy of offering a lowered professional fee for the procedure if the patient agrees to be a study participant, as patients may be required to make follow-up visits that may be time-consuming. Participating in studies can be used as a volume-building strategy.

The independent surgeons who do not compete on price and do not routinely discount fees are those with well-established reputations. Perhaps they participated in the manufacturers' clinical trials or began performing laser vision correction earlier than did most others. These are the early adopters, the doctors who had anticipated the introduction of the excimer laser long before the FDA approved it and have built a refractive practice from these early days.

These doctors have gained significant exposure within the professional community as a result, and many have a referral network in place. Consequently, they have the patient volume to support the cost of the laser. They also benefit from "word of mouth." Most refractive patients first consider laser surgery after someone they know has had the procedure. Satisfied patients make excellent ambassadors for whoever provided their treatment. Many of these physicians operate independently and have significantly less overhead than do the eye-care chains. They can charge considerably less and still make a handsome profit. Some do charge less, some don't.

In any case, so that you have some point of reference, you can expect to pay for PRK somewhere in the neighborhood of $2,000 per eye; for LASIK, $2,500; and for hyperopic LASIK, $2,750.

You Get What You Pay For

Because we all like to think we got the best deal for our money, we have a tendency to price-shop, even when it comes to something as important as our eyesight. We can't help it. So, when you are price-shopping, here are some things to consider.

First, in the end, poor medicine is no bargain. You might pay considerably less for the surgery and end up paying more in follow-up care with another doctor to treat resulting vision problems. If a provider is offering the procedure for significantly less than the going market rate, he or she has to be cutting costs somewhere or else has very deep pockets and hopes to make up in volume what is lost in per-case profit margins.

Where might these providers be cutting costs? On equipment: they might have the laser serviced less often than recommended and might replace damaged parts only when the laser actually stops as a result of failed parts. For the laser to perform optimally, the optics (the mirrors inside the machine that direct the laser beam along its path) must be changed according to a maintenance schedule. Optics are expensive to replace. Someone cutting corners might dispense with routine maintenance.

The doctor may be using a "gray market" laser. These are lasers once used in another country, shipped back to the United States, reconditioned, and sold at a much lower cost than is a new laser direct from the manufacturer. Or they could have a "black box" laser, which essentially is a "do-it-yourself" laser that is usually constructed by an engineer. Use of black box and gray market lasers doesn't necessarily result in poor outcomes, but the lasers probably have not passed the rigorous performance tests required by the FDA to be certified as safe and effective prior to commercial sale.

Some doctors using black box lasers also might do so with approval from the FDA in the form of an investigational device exemption (IDE). Doctors and/or treatment facilities can apply to the FDA for an exemption from restrictions against use of a medical device. They must submit to the agency how they will use the device, what safety precautions will be taken, how patients will be selected for treatment, precisely how that treatment will be administered, and how patients will be monitored during follow-up. This is called the study protocol. If an IDE is granted, then the doctor is free to use that device according to the protocol of his or her study. The FDA monitors this quite closely. (See chapter 10 for a comprehensive discussion of IDEs.) If you learn that the surgeon you are considering as your provider does not use an approved laser, you might want to ask if he or she has an IDE. If that person doesn't, you might want to consider a different surgeon.

Low-cost providers might also cut corners in usage and maintenance of other equipment. For example, the microkeratome is a delicate surgical instrument requiring careful cleaning, sterilization, and re-assembly between uses. To save money, it's possible that these providers have only one microkeratome, which costs between $50,000 and $75,000, and use it for a full day of procedures and forgo between-patient sterilization. This is much more common in South

America than in North America. The device also must periodically be shipped back to the manufacturer for inspection and repair of any damage that might have occurred to its gears or internal mechanisms. That level of maintenance can't be accomplished anywhere but at the factory, and each such inspection costs $1,500 or more, depending on necessary repairs. Waiting until the device fails, which can result in poor flaps and patients with unacceptable outcomes, can save a lot of money.

The microkeratome blade, at $50 apiece, is a fixed cost that can be made a variable cost if used on more than one patient. Reputable centers use one blade per patient to avoid infection and potential flap complications from a damaged or progressively dulled blade. The risk of both problems increases significantly the more times the blade is used.

Other ways that low-cost providers might cut costs is in staffing and staff training, using lesser-quality medical supplies and equipment, or using eyedrops and other medications past their expiration date. None of these things will necessarily result in a poor outcome for the patient, but why take that chance?

The microkeratome blade, at $50 apiece, is a fixed cost that can be made a variable cost if used on more than one patient. Reputable centers use one blade per patient to avoid infection and potential flap complications from a damaged or progressively dulled blade.

Elias Vamvakas, co-founder and CEO of TLC Laser Eye Centers, likens it to buying one car because it costs several thousand dollars less than another, without considering whether the car has air bags, anti-lock brakes, seat belts, or bumpers that can withstand impact because you don't believe that you'll ever be in an accident. Comments Mr. Vamvakas, "If you ever are in an accident, you're going to regret not buying the car with all the safety features. Going to a low-cost provider might save you a few hundred dollars on the procedure, but if something goes wrong you might regret not going to the provider who takes pains to ensure your safety and a good outcome."

Optometrist Jim Thimons suggests that when you compare costs, you might want to ask such questions as:

> What kind of laser do you use?
>
> How frequently is the laser serviced?
>
> When was the last time the microkeratome was sent to the manufacturer for reconditioning?
>
> Do you use the same microkeratome blade on multiple patients or do you change the blade between patients?

You may get some surprised looks and some doctors might be reluctant to answer those questions, but they certainly will know you've done your homework.

Comparing Apples to Apples

When comparing prices that are within a few hundred dollars of each other, make sure you're comparing apples to apples. Be direct. Ask the person who answers the phone at the center or at the surgeon's office what, exactly, the fee covers. Some procedures might look like bargains, but when you add up all the "extras," the cost is the same or more than a competitor's cost.

Questions to ask about cost include:

How much does the consultation and preoperative examination cost?

Many centers offer evaluations free of charge, whether the patient decides to have the procedure or not. Others charge the patient for the preoperative examination and then discount the procedure fee by that amount when the patient has surgery. These same facilities may charge for follow-up care separately.

Still others charge a separate fee for the consultation and preoperative exam. These same facilities also may charge separately for follow-up care. This strategy makes it appear as if the procedure cost is lower than a competitor's when, in fact, it isn't. If you add the costs together, they equal or exceed the amount charged by a center with a "global fee." Sometimes the manufacturer's royalty fee is added in after the price in the advertisement.

How much will I have to spend on postoperative medications and supplies?

Many centers provide patients with everything they will need postoperatively. For example, TLC's "post-op kit" contains wraparound sunglasses, individually wrapped Tylenol packets, eye shields, surgical tape for securing the shields, artificial tears to ease the discomfort of dry eyes, and small bottles of antibiotic and anti-inflammatory drops. The kit also contains written postoperative instructions that repeat the instructions given by the patient consultant at the center. Patients very likely will have to purchase artificial tears from the drugstore for several weeks, but they are not expensive. Some centers give the patient a prescription for eyedrops and pain medication, and patients are expected to buy them on their own.

How much will it cost if I have to have a second procedure?

Most centers and most independent physicians do not charge a fee for enhancements if performed within a specified period of time, usually a year. Retreatment, if needed, almost always is included in the original cost of the surgery.

But that is not a given, so it's important to ask. Also, some national chains now promise to provide no-cost enhancements for life, providing patients follow all postoperative instructions, including that they have the required follow-up examinations; have an annual eye exam to ensure continued good ocular health; and are medically suited to have another refractive procedure—in other words, there is sufficient corneal tissue remaining to safely perform another procedure and no other contraindication exists.

TLC was the first national laser vision correction company chain to offer what it calls its "Lifetime Commitment" program; others such as LCA Vision followed suit. These programs have stirred a degree of controversy among eye-care professionals, some of whom insist that they give the centers an unfair advantage over independents who can't afford to be so generous. Others say that the programs are thinly disguised attempts to guarantee referring optometrists a steady revenue stream.

The fact is, because refractive surgery is elective, providers have to work a whole lot harder to ensure patient satisfaction. The unwritten rule is that a happy patient tells ten people about how wonderful the procedure is, one or two of whom might then have the surgery themselves with the same doctors at the same facility. An unhappy patient tells 100 people, some of whom very likely are candidates for laser vision correction who will as a result put off the decision. Consequently, doctors work hard to ensure that every patient is a satisfied patient.

As hard as it is for some people to hear this, a lifetime commitment program is as much good marketing as it is good medicine. And there's nothing wrong with that. The marketing of medical procedures, products, and providers now is common practice. But this doesn't mean that having an annual eye exam is a bad idea. Your vision changes as you age. Many ocular health problems are asymptomatic, in that they can occur and cause damage before the patient is even aware that he or she has a problem. Particularly as we get older, annual eye exams, just like twice-yearly dental checkups, just make good sense.

Buyer Beware

The marketing of medicine is a fact of life, and it's becoming increasingly sophisticated. So, buyers beware; when listening to advertisements for a laser vision correction provider, do so with a caution. Although health-care providers have very specific guidelines they must follow and are closely monitored by the Federal Trade Commission (FTC) to ensure compliance, often advertising will "push the envelope," hoping to evade detection and censorship.

No advertiser can make false claims about a product, and medical advertisements are even more closely scrutinized than are others, for obvious reasons. However, that doesn't mean that false claims aren't made. They are.

> *No advertiser can make false claims about a product, and medical advertisements are even more closely scrutinized than are others, for obvious reasons. However, that doesn't mean that false claims aren't made. They are.*

Things to watch out for include blatant violations of truth in advertising, such as "Throw away your glasses and contacts forever," or images that suggest you will be rid of corrective lenses forever, such as a wastebasket filled with vision-care products. No one can guarantee you that you will not need corrective lenses after the procedure. You might need them only for reading or night driving. Or if you have a high degree of refractive error, you might have to continue to depend on corrective lenses for good vision, but the lenses won't be as strong as they once were.

Other deceptive claims may be "I was the first," "I've done more," "My results are the best." Only one doctor can claim this. Do your homework.

Advertisers also frequently make claims about a surgeon's level of experience with refractive surgery. Often you will hear on the radio or read in the newspaper that "Dr. X has performed several thousand refractive procedures." Don't believe everything you read or hear. A doctor can claim to have done several thousand refractive procedures and never have done a single PRK or LASIK procedure. They can because, technically, cataract surgery is a refractive procedure, and many, many doctors have done thousands of cataract surgeries. Doctors also may count RK in their refractive procedures. RK is a refractive procedure, to be sure, but it does not involve the excimer laser. So, having RK experience probably helps a surgeon gain a level of confidence with refractive surgery in general, but it does not make him or her a more experienced excimer laser refractive surgeon. It is a subtle but important difference.

When responding to an advertisement, ask the doctor or his or her staff how many excimer laser refractive procedures he or she has performed. Be even more specific. If you are considering LASIK, for example, ask the staff how many LASIK procedures the doctor has performed. Only then will you truly know how experienced or inexperienced the doctor is.

Laser vision correction advertisements cannot say that the procedure is painless, because there is a possibility that someone could experience some discomfort. There is no sensation of pain in the cornea because it is anesthetized, but some patients do feel discomfort around the area where the eyelid speculum rests against the brow.

They cannot make any claims about results unless they have, and reference, verifiable statistical data. As there is no requirement that surgeons maintain or report outcome data, most advertisers use data gathered during the clinical trials (which, typically, the doctors did not participate in). This is unfortunate because the clinical trial data are old and the data just keep getting better. The best surgeons do compile their own data to monitor their own outcomes and to help their nomograms (the formula they use to program desired correction into the laser). So, as was suggested in an earlier chapter, if you're interested ask the surgeon if you can see his or her outcome data. Most of them will be happy to share it with you.

Furthermore, neither laser manufacturers, laser-center owners, nor physicians can advertise the use of the laser in a treatment for which it has not been approved. Doctors were permitted to perform LASIK before the lasers were approved for use in LASIK because it was considered a "practice of medicine" issue—something to be decided between the doctor and the patient—but they could not advertise use of the laser for that purpose. (See chapter 10.) However, in July 1999 the FDA Ophthalmic Advisory Panel recommended approval of the VISX and Summit Technology lasers for use in LASIK. Should the FDA follow the panel's recommendation and approve the lasers for use in LASIK, both the manufacturers and users of the device will be able to advertise that LASIK is an available treatment option.

Reputable facilities adhere to these guidelines because it is in the best interests of the patient. Large, corporately owned chains have attorneys on staff who ensure compliance with federal and state guidelines regarding medical marketing. Failing to do so could result in severe financial penalties. Independents may not be as well versed in the finer points of FTC regulations, but all of them are aware of the standards and practices established by their own profession. There is no excuse for deceptive advertising.

Advertisers use lots of "patient friendly" words to make refractive surgery sound less frightening. Almost all emphasize that the laser beam is from the "cool" end of the light spectrum, which it is. Many refer to the corneal cap as a protective flap, which is "created" rather than "sliced" or "cut." In advertisements and commercials for laser vision correction you will hear or read such words as *gentle, quick, fast-healing,* and *forever.*

You might even hear or read that LASIK and PRK are noninvasive procedures. This is a bit over the line. PRK is not incisional—a knife is not used to cut into the tissue—but it is invasive. LASIK is both incisional and invasive. Surgery is by its nature invasive. In LASIK and PRK, human tissue is disrupted and a wound is created, and that's invasive.

Much of what you read and hear will be true, technically, but remember, it is marketing. We recommend you make your decision based on the facts, not the hype. As with the marketing of any product or service, the best caution for those considering laser vision correction is buyer beware.

Fee for Service

Although laser vision correction centers structure financial reimbursements differently, generally speaking, patients are paying a facility fee, a professional fee to the surgeon, and a professional fee for pre- and postoperative care, if the doctor providing that care is other than the surgeon. How much of the total fee is distributed where depends entirely on the facility, the physician, who's providing care, and where that care is provided. Confusing, yes?

Usually, for the patient's convenience, a "global" payment is collected before the procedure is performed and the funds are distributed appropriately by the facility administrator. Some facilities ask patients to write out separate checks for each.

Here's another way to think of it. If you were to have knee surgery at an outpatient facility, you would be asked to pay a facility fee, a fee to the anesthesiologist, a fee to the radiologist, one to the surgeon, and another to the referring doctor, your personal physician, if that doctor provided follow-up care. The outpatient facility where you have your surgery might be a management company that collects a global fee as a convenience to you, the patient, and takes responsibility for disbursing funds to the other parties involved in your care. This often happens, but usually insurance pays so you are not aware of how the funds are distributed. It's no different with laser vision correction, except that probably a third party won't later cover the check you write.

Co-managing patients is common practice in many fields of medicine. As you remember, in chapter 4 we discussed the co-management of laser vision correction patients. In refractive surgery, co-management is an arrangement whereby one doctor, usually an optometrist but sometimes a general ophthalmologist who prefers not to do LASIK, provides patients with the preoperative consultation and examination and with postoperative care, and refers the patient to a refractive surgeon for the surgery. Fees for those services are paid accordingly.

In the course of researching laser vision correction, you will most likely come across articles and items on the Internet that refer to the co-management of patients and hint of something slightly sinister. There is nothing sinister about it. Medical professionals refer patients to other medical specialists all the time. Each is paid for whatever services are provided.

More attention is paid to co-management of laser vision correction patients because the procedure is becoming widespread—"commercialized"—and because, historically, the relationship between optometrists and ophthalmologists has been strained. This tension results from the fact that optometrists recently have been approved to provide care that also is within an ophthalmologist's likely range of medical services, particularly a general ophthalmologist's. At the time of publication, optometrists can't perform surgery in any state.

A lingering fear among optometrists is that if they refer their patients to an ophthalmologist for refractive surgery or for any other surgical procedure or ocular health concern, that patient will never return to their practice, nor will any potential patient referrals accrue to the optometrist. A patient referred to a refractive surgeon is potentially a lost patient. And that's at the heart of the controversy. In fact, most high-volume surgeons would prefer not to spend their time in routine, uneventful patient follow-up because it takes time away from their surgical practice. You will quickly learn that virtually all busy refractive surgeons have an optometrist on their staff on whom they rely for pre- and post-op care. So, now you know what all the fuss is about.

Insurance Coverage

If you plan to have laser vision correction, plan to pay for it yourself. Some, but not many, insurance companies do pay some of the costs. Of course, it doesn't hurt to ask, but don't be surprised if the company says no. And don't be surprised if the representative who answers the telephone at your insurance company has no idea what you're talking about when you ask if the company covers LASIK, PRK, or refractive surgery.

Bill Leonard, vice president of operations with TLC, explains: "Not a lot of insurance companies cover refractive surgery. Those that do are usually self-funded plans such as the ones offered by United Parcel Service, some unions, and Honda Motors, and coverage changes daily. Most such plans require the patient to pay 20 percent of the total cost. Also, many plans that started out paying for the procedure stopped doing so when they learned how many people were eligible and anxious to have laser vision correction. It became too expensive.

> *Some, but not many, insurance companies do pay some of the costs. Of course, it doesn't hurt to ask, but don't be surprised if the company says no.*

"Interestingly, some insurance companies do cover RK or ALK, but don't cover PRK or LASIK, or if they do, they do so at a greatly reduced rate. This probably is because there are insurance codes for the former, but not for the latter."

Insurance companies make a distinction between functional surgery and cosmetic surgery. Functional surgery is that which is intended to treat a disease or health condition that would otherwise progress. Cancer surgery is functional surgery. Hip replacement surgery is functional surgery. Removal of a brain tumor is functional surgery; so is removal of a cataract. Leaving a cataract can lead to functional blindness. Surgery that is not functional is cosmetic, meaning it is intended solely to change a person's physical appearance or some external feature of the body.

Cosmetic surgery is divided into two categories: that which is intended to correct a disfigurement caused by birth defect, disease, or accident; and that which is intended to improve the patient's general appearance. Insurance pays for the former but not for the latter. Insurance carriers also cover cosmetic surgery that is deemed medically necessary. Sometimes there is overlap between that which is intended to correct some defect and that which improves one's general appearance.

Some refractive surgery patients have successfully argued that point in court. One man claimed that his extremely high myopia was, in fact, a handicap, and, therefore, his insurance carrier should pay for the correction of that handicap. The court ruled in his favor, but no one recommends people take that approach. It's expensive, for one thing, and it isn't likely to have the same outcome. You may feel handicapped by your refractive error, and in many ways you are, but it probably will be difficult to persuade your insurance carrier of that.

It's hard to say if insurance companies ever will cover laser vision correction. Elias Vamvakas believes that ultimately, the procedure will be included in a company's menu of benefits just as contact lenses and eyeglasses are now; that companies offering vision-care plans will incorporate refractive surgery into those plans. Some already do. Some companies now pay $200 or more a year toward the cost of an employee's eye-care and will contribute that amount toward the cost of refractive surgery. That's probably a fairly safe prediction.

To be perfectly honest, most doctors and probably most treatment centers would prefer that insurance not cover the procedure. Historically, when third-party payers get involved, the treatment and facility fees plummet. That certainly has been true with reimbursements for cataract surgery.

There is a lot of speculation now that the cost of laser vision correction will drop precipitously over the next few years, as the technology gets cheaper and more competitors enter the market. Don't count on it. That has not been the trend in cosmetic surgery or orthodontia, the only two areas of elective medicine that are in any way comparable. And in fact, in some markets, the procedure price has actually gone up with the introduction of LASIK and a treatment for hyperopia.

There also is speculation that doctors not only don't want insurance to cover the procedure, but that they refer and treat refractive patients with no regard for what is in the patient's best interests, to recover revenues lost to lowered reimbursements for cataract surgery. Doctors have lost income due to lowered reimbursements, but no reputable doctor would recommend a procedure to a patient for whom the treatment was inappropriate. As was said in the previous chapter, it isn't good medicine and it isn't good business.

Payment Plans

There are ways to make the procedure more affordable. All management companies and most independent doctors and practices offer some kind of payment plan. A number of financial services companies specialize in making funds available for nonreimbursable procedures. The terms and conditions vary widely. Some are "like cash," in that no interest is charged if the full amount is paid back within ninety days; others allow patients to pay over twenty-four to thirty-six months.

Most centers and many doctors accept major credit cards, and some surgeons offer what amounts to a "no-interest" loan to qualifying patients. To learn more about payment plans, call a laser vision correction center in your area and ask to speak with a patient consultant.

Laser vision correction also is tax-deductible as a medical expense and can be paid for with pre-tax dollars set aside in your company-administered Flexible Benefits Plan. Some people have paid for the procedure with a home equity loan, the interest on which is tax-deductible. If you are considering such a payment plan, you might want to first speak with your tax adviser. The point is, cost is not as much of an issue as you might think.

What Am I Willing to Pay?

As you make your decision about laser vision correction, you might want to turn around the original question, What can I expect to pay? Ask instead, What am I willing to pay? How much am I willing to pay to reduce my dependence on, or eliminate my need for, eyeglasses and contact lenses? What will I pay to receive care from the most experienced surgeon in my area who offers me the greatest chance of achieving the best possible outcome. When it comes to the cost of the procedure, that's the only question that really matters. Whether or not your insurance carrier will pay all or some of the cost now or sometime in the future is secondary.

When Dr. Machat talks to other doctors about building a refractive practice, he often whimsically comments, "I've never, ever had a patient come to me after surgery and say, 'Gee, doc, my vision is great, but I think you charged too much.'" When the benefits are apparent, cost becomes less of an issue. Whether you can afford it or not is an issue, but how much it costs becomes less important. Only you know the value you put on a life without corrective lenses or with lenses for only certain tasks like reading or night driving. Only you know if this is something on which you would choose to spend your discretionary income.

For many reasons, who makes money from health care has become an extremely controversial, emotionally charged issue, but it doesn't have to be. Health care is a business, like all other businesses. Emotion comes in because the business involves a person's well-being. Take the emotion out and it's possible to appreciate laser vision correction for what it is, a treatment that can improve a person's quality of life, job prospects, and self-confidence.

So, before you answer the question What am I willing to pay? maybe it would help to understand a little bit about the business of medicine in general, and of refractive surgery specifically.

Remember, Medicine Is a Business

And it is potentially a big business, just as is all health-care delivery. In recent years, specialty health clinics have become a much larger component of the health-care delivery sector. There are specialty clinics for life-threatening or life-compromising conditions such as heart disease and cancer. And there are specialty clinics that cater to the desire in all of us to look and feel better. These include hair-replacement clinics; weight loss centers; holistic health facilities providing chiropractic care, acupuncture, biofeedback, and the like; cosmetic surgery centers; and, more recently, laser vision correction centers.

Fewer and fewer of us receive any but emergency or major medical treatment in a hospital setting, and more of us are paying out of pocket for the specialized care we need or want. There's nothing inherently wrong with that. It's just that Americans are used to having someone else foot the bill for medical products and procedures.

For decades, third-party payers such as private insurance companies, usually subsidized by employers and the government, have paid whatever fee-for-service was set by the health profession, no questions asked. This brought the United States as close to socialized medicine as our democratic society has ever come. The altruistic goal was universal access to first-rate, affordable health care. While this was never quite reached, the country came close, and often the patient paid nothing.

Managed Care Changed Everything

As you know, managed care changed everything—not always for the better, many would argue. But perhaps most important, it introduced into a historically poorly managed industry such business concepts as economies of scale, consistency of service, and cost-cutting. Medicine was introduced to marketing. Doctors, hospitals, specialty clinics, and even pharmaceutical companies began advertising, first within the profession, but shortly thereafter direct to consumers. The health-care industry underwent dramatic changes.

Although managed care was once embraced as the solution to skyrocketing health-care costs, now a growing cadre of activists believe that it has failed. All the "fat" that could have been cut out of the health-care delivery system has been cut and now quality of care is taking a backseat to profitability. As resentment toward HMOs grows, a vociferous national debate has ignited in regard to all health-care costs: Who pays, how much, for what, and who profits have become cocktail party chatter.

Providers of laser vision correction quite naturally are part of that debate for a number of reasons. The procedure is new, it's elective, and it's expensive. Furthermore, most insurance companies don't cover the costs. (Well, as you learned in the first chapter, it isn't exactly new, but the public has become more aware of it lately and it is more widely available.) Because the technology is expensive and the cost of operating a laser vision correction facility is high, there is a procedure "price point" below which most laser centers cannot go and still remain viable.

> *As resentment toward HMOs grows, a vociferous national debate has ignited in regard to all health-care costs: Who pays, how much, for what, and who profits have become cocktail party chatter.*

Introduce into the controversy the fact that, historically, there has been tension between the two eye-care professions, ophthalmology and optometry, which provides fertile ground for the seeds of discontent from which grow rumor and innuendo.

Millions Invested—Altruism or Profit Motive?

People are making money from refractive surgery. Executives and investors in health-care businesses often do make a lot of money, but not before they've invested a lot of money and time in the development of products and services. And, yes, many doctors make a lot of money. But that should not be relevant to your decision about having the procedure or how much you're willing to pay.

Think of it this way: Bill Gates has more money than anyone else in the world, yet just about all of us have purchased a Microsoft product in the past few years, perhaps without even being aware of it. Few of us would decide not to buy a computer or a software program because it might mean that Bill Gates would make a few more dollars.

The excimer laser was in development for more than a decade before it was approved for commercial sale. Millions and millions of dollars were spent to perfect the technology and the technique and to demonstrate to the FDA's satisfaction that the device was safe and effective for use in humans. As laser manufacturers, investors, and individuals poured millions into a promise that might never pay off, more millions were being spent by entrepreneurs such as Gary Jonas, founder of 20/20 Laser Centers; Elias Vamvakas, founder and CEO of TLC, which now owns 20/20; Steve Joffee, M.D., CEO of Laser Centers of America; and Donald Wingerter, Jr., president and CEO of Clear Vision. Their goal was to figure out the most efficient and most cost-effective way to make the procedure available to the greatest number of people.

There were many more whose companies didn't make it to the point of approval of the excimer laser or that failed just afterward. They didn't make it because they ran out of money before money could be earned from the procedure or because they had the wrong business model. Some, like 20/20 Laser Centers, didn't make it on their own because a larger or wealthier company acquired them.

In any case, anticipating a return on investment is how all business works. The development of the excimer laser can be compared to the development of "blockbuster" drugs such as Prozac, Valium, and Viagra. Pharmaceutical companies identify conditions for which the potential treatment market is large and spend millions to develop products that treat those conditions. For their efforts, they often are handsomely rewarded. Pfizer, for example, hit pay dirt with the development of Viagra, the anti-impotence drug. It's expected to be an $11-billion-a-year market.

Are those involved in health care inspired by altruism or by the profit motive? Both, to be honest. But that isn't the only thing that motivates people in the industry. That they can bring so much joy to so many is a powerful motivating force. How many of us go to work knowing that at the end of the day, we will have improved the quality of life for hundreds, maybe thousands of people?

Companies like TLC, LCA Vision, Clear Vision, and others have contributed more than just dollars to the development of laser vision correction. Through the efforts of such companies, people throughout the country are being educated about the procedure and are being given the opportunity to decide for themselves whether refractive surgery is right for them.

In fact, it was 20/20 Laser Centers that coined the term *laser vision correction*. Early in the company's development Gary Jonas realized that *photorefractive keratectomy* was not a term that most people would respond well to. It was too hard to say and not nearly descriptive enough. At a company-wide strategy session, he challenged those of us at the meeting to come up with a word or phrase that would describe the procedure and that patients would be able to understand without using a medical dictionary. The group came up with *laser vision correction* and began using the term in all of its patient education materials. That same year, VISX and Summit both used the term in their annual reports. Now it is in the public domain. It is the way everyone refers to this remarkable vision correction alternative.

A myth taking shape in cyberspace is that corporate-owned laser centers are more concerned with patient volume and earning a profit than they are with quality of care given to patients. Nothing could be further from the truth. Any businessperson can tell you that if the care isn't high quality, eventually there will be no patient volume and no profits.

As Dr. Brint, Dr. Kennedy, and I have said several times before, it's your decision and yours alone. Don't let anyone talk you into or out of having laser vision correction. Only you know if you can afford it, and only you know if it's right for you.

9

Should I Wait Until the Technology Gets Better?

In an earlier chapter I recounted a story that Dr. Jeffery Machat enjoys repeating when people ask him if they should wait to have laser vision correction. He tells them of a friend on whom he performed refractive surgery nearly seven years ago. The man had an uneventful surgery, was corrected to 20/15 in both eyes, and experienced no complications. His vision, in other words, was excellent.

However, on a return visit a few years later he saw that Dr. Machat had a new laser. Upon receiving a positive response to his question: Is this a better laser? Dr. Machat's friend shrugged his shoulders regretfully and said, "Gosh, I should have waited."

About which Dr. Machat wryly asks, "How do you respond to a comment like that? Waited for what? How much better does he think his vision would have been if he had waited?"

That's the point that Dr. Mark Whitten makes when patients ask him that question. He tells them that for most people, the technology available today is as good as it needs to be to give them excellent results. But, he adds:

"There are some people who should wait. People with corneas that are too thin, pupils that are too large, or refractive errors that are too high (greater than −15.00 or +6.00) should wait. Also, people with irregular or unusual astigmatism should wait because there are lasers in development that will give them better results."

He reminds patients not to think just about the technology but about their own needs, and uses himself as an example. Says Dr. Whitten: "In 1995, I went to Canada and had PRK to correct my refractive error of −5.00 in both eyes. That afternoon I was on the golf course. Today, I am 20/15 in one eye and 20/20 in the other. For me, for my level of correction, the technology was as good as it needed to be. I don't think I would have gotten a substantially better result if I had waited. And that was in 1995, when LASIK was just being developed. Already, today, the technology and the technique are light-years ahead of where they were when I had PRK."

Elias Vamvakas, CEO of TLC Laser Eye Centers, and Dr. Machat both make a comparison to computers and other electronic equipment. Lots of us have purchased, or soon will purchase, a personal computer even though we know the technology will get better. We know that in the future computers will be more powerful, the graphics crisper and more realistic, and the computing capabilities greater, but the benefits of having one now outweigh the risk of obsolescence. Similarly, few of us would decide not to buy a television set today even though we know that sometime in the next few years high-definition television will make whatever we now own obsolete.

In reality, most of us buy the best available product, providing it meets our current needs. If everyone waited for perfection, we all would still be tapping away at a typewriter while listening to the radio.

Of course, there's a big difference between electronic equipment and eye surgery, but the point is well taken. The truth is that the technology used in refractive surgery and the techniques used to ensure a good outcome get better every day. Already, Summit and VISX, the two manufacturers that have had FDA approval the longest (since October 1995 and March 1996, respectively) are producing third-generation lasers. They're working constantly to obtain a smoother ablation and a wider treatment zone and to influence any part of the human healing response that can be affected by laser beam delivery.

> *In reality, most of us buy the best available product, providing it meets our current needs. If everyone waited for perfection, we all would still be tapping away at a typewriter while listening to the radio.*

Other laser manufacturers, including Autonomous Technologies, now a division of Summit Technology (LADARSystem approved for use in PRK up to −10.00 diopters); LaserSight; Nidek (approved for use in PRK up to −13.00 diopters); and Bausch & Lomb Surgical (now approved for use in PRK to treat nearsightedness) are developing lasers with different beam profiles and different delivery paths. Some have tracking systems that enable the laser to follow the eye's every movement to ensure proper correction even if the patient moves inadvertently. Down the road are topography-assisted lasers, which means that the laser beam can be directed to follow the precise contours of the cornea by following a computerized map created by a corneal topographer. (See chapter 6 for a description of corneal topography.)

Explains Dr. Whitten, "Today, our goal is to give patients the best possible vision, but we can't make it better than it was before surgery. We can make it as good as it was with contact lenses or eyeglasses, but we can't make it better. With corneal topography–assisted lasers we may be able to make people's vision better than it was before because we will be able to identify and remove tiny, naturally occurring surface irregularities, which will improve their quality of vision as well as visual acuity."

Eric Ankerud, vice president of regulatory clinical affairs with Summit Technology, says that the industry is headed toward customized corneas. In July 1999, Summit's subsidiary, Autonomous Technologies, received an investigational device exemption (IDE) from the FDA to begin clinical trials of its proprietary CustomCornea in combination with its already approved LADARVision System, to test the safety and effectiveness of topography-assisted laser treatments. (See chapter 10 for a discussion of IDEs.)

Eric Donnenfeld, M.D., a refractive surgeon in Nassau County, Long Island, New York, says the next step in laser technology will result in "designer eyes." One day surgeons will select precisely how good to make your near vision and how good to make your far vision to enable you to have the best possible vision given your lifestyle, profession, and personality. Irregular surfaces will be smoothed to give the best quality vision possible. Of course, the technology isn't there yet, but it's getting close.

Researchers around the country also are experimenting with techniques that have nothing to do with the excimer laser. Included among them are intracorneal rings (recently approved for low myopia, up to −3.00 diopters), contact lens implants, and lens replacements, which would entail removing the crystalline lens and replacing it with a permanent plastic lens. Today, this is commonly done to treat cataracts.

Considerable energy is being devoted to improving the microkeratome, the device used to create the corneal flap. There are, at last count, eighteen companies hoping to make the next big breakthrough in microkeratome technology and in the process capture some of the market now dominated by Bausch & Lomb's Automated Corneal Shaper and its newer model, the Hansatome. The Hansatome creates a larger corneal flap and is preferred by most refractive surgeons for the treatment of hyperopia.

LaserSight Technologies, for example, markets a disposable microkeratome that comes fully assembled in a sterile packet. It's called the Automated Disposable Keratome and is said to reduce the risk of complications resulting from improper device assembly and the risk of infection from improperly cleaned equipment. Others are developing devices that create the corneal flap with a high-speed jet of water or with a solid-state laser. Presumed safety advantages would be reduced risk of debris under the corneal cap and the creation of flaps with smoother edges, reducing the risk of epithelial ingrowth.

If your refractive error puts you in the elite company of the fewer than 5 percent of the lens-wearing population who would do well to wait, read on. Or read on if you're just curious to know what will be possible in the next few years with lasers and with other refractive techniques.

How Lasers Work

The word *laser,* as you might recall from high school physics and from chapter 1, is an acronym for "light amplification by the stimulated emission of radiation."

Visible light is a form of electromagnetic radiation. There are other forms as well: x-rays and radio waves, for example. Each carries energy. Every form of electromagnetic radiation can be made to interact with another. When an interaction is forced, energy is released and light is produced.

Lasers are a method of producing an intense beam of energy with a precise wavelength, or color. The "lasing effect" is achieved when atoms, which exist at low and high energy levels, are excited to greater levels of activity, sometimes by heating but also by being bombarded by light of a higher frequency or stimulated by electricity. On reaching higher levels and then returning to lower levels, atoms give off light.

Atoms in any substance—gases, liquids, organic dyes, rare-earth elements such as rubies and sapphires, and certain chemical compounds are among the substances used in laser technology—emit light independently and in many different colors, or wavelengths. During the brief time an atom is excited, if light of a certain color impinges on it, the atom can be stimulated to emit radiation. The radiation amplifies the light.

If the phenomenon is multiplied—that is, if all the atoms are excited to the same level of energy—the resulting beam, made up of wholly coherent light of a single color, will be extremely powerful. Using conventional lens systems (optics), that light can be focused on a specific spot. Whether a laser beam is beneficial or harmful depends on the wavelength of the energy source, the strength of the radiation, and the substances with which it interacts. Light that comes from the higher end of the ultraviolet spectrum generates intense heat. Light from the lower end of the spectrum generates lesser amounts of heat.

In the excimer laser a mixture of argon and fluoride gases, called dimers, is excited by electricity (excited + dimer = excimer) to emit radiation at a wavelength of 193.3 nanometers (nm). The excimer laser was a revolutionary breakthrough for refractive surgery. Unlike other lasers used in various types of surgery, the excimer laser generates sufficient energy to excite molecules to the point of separation but not enough energy to burn through and damage surrounding tissue.

It's called a "cool" laser, because it generates light at the lower end of the ultraviolet spectrum. The excimer laser removes tissue through a process called photoablation, which entails bombarding molecules with light to the point of separation. The molecules are vaporized rather than exploded or burned, as they would be using a laser that relied on thermal energy (heat generation). And remember, we're talking about removing tissue in fractions of microns—0.25 microns for each pulse of the laser, to be precise. Furthermore, after each laser pulse the remaining tissue cell is resealed by the formation of a new membrane.

Unlike other lasers used in various types of surgery, the excimer laser generates sufficient energy to excite molecules to the point of separation but not enough energy to burn through and damage surrounding tissue.

As noted previously in the book, the cornea is typically between 500 and 600 microns thick. It would take 2,000 pulses to go through the cornea. A strand of hair is about 125 microns thick; it would take 500 excimer laser pulses to break the strand. In refractive surgery, surgeons remove anywhere from 10 to 160 microns of tissue so the laser beam doesn't come close to penetrating the cornea.

Improvements in the Laser

The physics of the laser are very complex and a detailed explanation is probably more than most of us want. Those who desire to know more should contact the laser manufacturers listed in the resource section in the back of the book.

But, basically, inside the high tech–looking piece of equipment is a chamber in which the gases are mixed and excited to create the lasing effect. A series of mirrors and prisms (called optics) reflects the light back and forth within the cavity to maintain that effect. The optics also direct a portion of the laser beam through the system and into the laser tube, which is directly over a patient's head and wherein is the red or green fixation light.

A diaphragm, or aperture, within the laser tube controls the size of the beam, where the beam hits the cornea, and for how long. When the laser technician programs your desired correction into the laser's computer, the computer determines the size, pattern, and duration of the laser treatment and adjusts the diaphragm accordingly.

There are basically two types of excimer lasers in use or in development, broad beam and scanning. These types refer to how the laser beam is delivered to the corneal surface. A broad beam gives a continuous flow of energy to the center of the cornea and outward, the flow controlled by the widening of the diaphragm, or aperture. Scanning lasers are either slit scanning or "flying spot." Both have smaller beams, 1 mm to 2 mm, that move around the cornea in a random but organized pattern.

It's too soon to know whether one delivers better results than the other, although the theory is that the scanning and "flying spot" lasers will create smoother ablations, which will result in a better quality of vision for the patient. As mentioned earlier, for the surgeon to achieve the best possible vision the corneal surface must be as smooth as possible. In the early days, broad beam lasers tended to create very subtle gradations in treatment areas, sort of like stairsteps, which might have caused some patients to experience glare or halos for longer than they might have if the surface were smoother.

The first two lasers to be approved for use in PRK were manufactured by VISX Inc. and Summit Technology. Both are broad beam lasers. Since then, VISX has introduced its SmoothScan technology, in which a broad beam is split into seven small-diameter beams that move across the cornea. And according to VISX, the SmoothScan system, in use in the VISX Star2, softens the image of the iris diaphragm edges, thereby eliminating rough edges and uneven transitions.

The other three lasers approved for use in PRK are the Nidek EC-5000, which is a scanning slit, Autonomous Technologies's laser, which is a "flying spot" laser, and LaserSight Technologies's laser, also a flying spot. The Autonomous laser also employs eye-tracking technology that enables the laser beam to follow the movements of a patient's eye, thereby eliminating the possibility of a decentered ablation resulting from undetected, involuntary movements. The eye-tracking technology is the same technology used in missile tracking. It was developed by Autonomous Technologies for the military as part of the Strategic Defense Initiative (Star Wars). In 1994, Autonomous formed an alliance with CIBA Vision. In 1999, Autonomous was acquired by Summit Technology.

Another important improvement that was made in all currently available lasers and those in development is the size of the treatment zone. Early lasers had apertures that only opened to 5.0 mm. If they were used on patients with large pupils, the treatment zone was smaller than the patient's optical zone when the pupil was fully dilated. One result was a pronounced and persistent glare as light entered the eye beyond the corrected area. These lasers also were not useful in the treatment of hyperopia, during which tissue is removed from the periphery of the optical zone to effectively make the cornea steeper. The smaller treatment zone did not provide the technology to go out farther in the 7-mm to 9-mm range to remove peripheral corneal tissue to correct hyperopia.

Every laser manufacturer is developing machines with larger treatment zones, most opening to 9 mm or 10 mm, which is sufficient for hyperopic treatment. The wider optical zone will also make it possible to create a smoother transition from the treatment zone to untreated corneal tissue, which will reduce incidence of glare and halos, particularly for people with higher levels of myopia and large pupils.

Topography-Assisted Lasers

Generating the most excitement among refractive sur-geons is the advent of corneal topography–assisted abla-tions: customized corneas. As described in chapter 5, dur-ing the preoperative examination, and often on the day of surgery, a technician takes a picture of your eye with a device called a corneal topographer, also called a video-keratographer. The computer-generated map shows the surgeon where your cornea is steepest, where there are surface irregularities, and the axis on which your astigma-tism is located, if you have astigmatism. Your surgeon uses the map as a guide when making decisions about your desired correction.

In the future, during treatment the laser will be guided by a corneal topographer that is mapping your eye and directing the laser beam according to where your cornea is steepest or where naturally occurring irregularities exist. If those irregularities are removed, the result will be improved quality and quantity of vision (visual acuity).

As David Eldridge, O.D., executive vice president of clinical affairs with TLC Laser Eye Centers, explains: "If you have five people all with refractive errors of −5.00 diopters, their prescriptions might be the same, but their corneal topographies would look very different. All the lit-tle irregularities would show up, those things that maybe compromise their night vision or affect their contrast sensitivity. With today's lasers, you can only program in a −5.00 diopters desired correction. There's nothing you can do about the more subtle surface irregularities. With corneal topography–assisted ablations, the surgeon will tell the laser's computer just exactly which segment of the corneal surface to change and by how much. Customized ablations will give people better vision with-out lenses than they had with them, unless they wore rigid gas-permeable lenses."

Holmium Lasers

Another laser you may have come across in your research into laser vision correction is the Holmium YAG laser, developed by Sunrise Technologies. The Ophthalmic Device Advisory Panel did not recommend that the FDA approve this laser at the July 1999 panel hearing. However, the manufacturer remains confident that laser thermal keratoplasty (LTK) will eventually be an approved alternative to excimer laser surgery for the treatment of low degrees of hyperopia and for PRK and LASIK hyperopic retreatments necessitated by overcorrection of myopia and for the treatment of presbyopia.

In LTK, heat is applied to the surface of the cornea to shrink the collagen fibers in a circular pattern around the periphery of the optical zone. The ring of contracted collagen creates a constrictive band, which forces the corneal tissue inside the band to bulge. The procedure takes only seconds and is considerably cheaper than excimer laser treatments. However, it is only effective in treating hyperopia up to +2.5 and patient's refractive error tends to regress in the first three to six months. The holmium is in limited use in Canada for the treatment of eyes overcorrected during PRK.

> *The problem with LTK has been determining how much heat to apply in how many locations to achieve desired results, and ensuring stability of results. These rather significant problems have yet to be solved.*

Research is ongoing as to whether LTK will prove useful as a treatment for presbyopia, particularly for people with no previous refractive error. Surgeons could induce monovision by changing the refraction on one eye to make it nearsighted for up-close vision and leaving the other untreated for distance vision.

Like LASIK, LTK has been in development for nearly a century. Physicians have known for some time that applying heat to the corneal surface would cause the collagen fibers to constrict and force a steepening of the cornea. The problem with LTK has been determining how much heat to apply in how many locations to achieve desired results, and ensuring stability of results. These rather significant problems have yet to be solved.

Refractive Techniques Without Lasers

A number of refractive surgical techniques are in development that do not involve the excimer laser. Included among these is a device called an intrastromal corneal ring and another called an implantable intraocular contact lens, also described as a phakic refractive IOL. *Phakia* means lens; *IOL* stands for intraocular lens. The aphakic IOL is used routinely to correct aphakia—the absence of the cloudy lens (the cataract). There are three techniques being studied for use of implantable refractive intraocular lenses in refractive surgery, each of which will be discussed shortly.

Corneal rings are effective for people with low degrees of myopia, up to −3.00 diopters. Implants, on the other hand, are considered more appropriate for people with higher degrees of refractive error, above −10.00 diopters or +6.00 diopters.

Corneal Ring

In April 1999, the FDA approved for commercial sale the Intacs corneal ring, manufactured by KeraVision, for use in people with myopic refractive errors up to −3.00 diopters and with less than 1.00 diopter of astigmatism. Intacs are tiny plastic arches that are implanted in the layer of the cornea called the stroma. The plastic used is the same bio-medical grade material that has been used for years in contact lenses and to make intraocular lens implants for the treatment of cataracts.

In a five- to fifteen-minute procedure, the surgeon makes a small (1.8 mm) incision in the cornea just outside the optical zone. As in LASIK, a suction ring is used, which holds the eye steady and gives the surgeon the largest possible corneal surface to work with. Using a specially designed surgical instrument, the stroma is separated to create a semicircular tunnel within the cornea. First one arch is inserted and rotated into position, then the second.

As with PRK and LASIK, there are advantages and disadvantages to corneal rings as a treatment for refractive errors. Arguably, the biggest advantage is that the procedure is reversible. A surgeon can always remove the rings if the patient is not happy with the results. Literature distributed by KeraVision also cites as a big advantage over laser vision correction that no corneal tissue is removed to accomplish the correction. That's true, but it is also true that the incision made in the cornea to accommodate the rings penetrates deeper (two-thirds the depth of the cornea) than does the laser ablation (up to one-third the depth of the cornea). Consequently, there is some risk of perforating the cornea.

Corneal rings have associated with them many of the same potential postsurgical complications as do PRK and LASIK, such as infection, glare, halos, overcorrection, undercorrection, double vision, induced astigmatism, fluctuating vision, and loss of best corrected visual acuity (BCVA). During clinical trials, incidence of these were in the range of 1 percent, a similar rate to their occurrence in laser vision correction.

According to Dr. Machat, a significant disadvantage of the corneal rings is that corrections can only be made in one-half diopters, whereas excimer lasers currently in use can be programmed to one-quarter of a diopter. Lasers now in clinical trials will be programmable to less than one-tenth a diopter of correction. In patients with low degrees of refractive error, one-half a diopter can make a significant difference in visual acuity, particularly since corrective lenses probably give them excellent vision. Corneal rings also cannot currently be used to treat astigmatism.

According to an article in *Ocular Surgery News,* a medical publication for ophthalmologists, corneal rings show promise for patients with low degrees of myopia who also have keratoconus, which is a disease of the cornea that causes it to grow thinner and steeper. Contact lenses and eyeglasses are the usual treatments for this condition. However, some patients become contact lens–intolerant, or their condition is such that contact lenses no longer improve their visual acuity. Eventually, these patients require a corneal transplant. In at least one study, six such patients received corneal ring implants, which were well tolerated and improved their vision, forestalling the need for a transplant.

At least at the time of this writing, most high-volume refractive surgeons consider the corneal rings a limited tool in the refractive surgery arsenal but nonetheless useful in some cases.

Implantable Contact Lens

Without a doubt, the most common ophthalmic surgery performed in the United States today is cataract surgery. More than 90 percent of these procedures involve the replacement of the crystalline lens, which has become cloudy, with an intraocular lens (IOL), also called aphakic IOL. Before the IOL was developed, the surgical treatment for cataracts entailed the removal of the crystalline lens. Without the crystalline lens, the eye cannot focus and patients would be forced to wear extremely thick glasses or contact lenses to correct their vision. An eye without the crystalline lens is said to be aphakic. Once the crystalline lens has been replaced by a man-made lens, the eye is said to be pseudophakic (false lens).

The introduction of the aphakic IOL gave surgeons the tool they needed to restore a cataract patient's vision. The IOL that is inserted is similar to a contact lens, in that it corrects for the loss of refractive power resulting from the removal of the crystalline lens. The amount of focusing power to be given a patient is determined by measuring the length of the eye and the curvature of the cornea. The length of the eye is measured with an ultrasound probe much like that used to obtain a sonogram of a fetus. That data is programmed into a computer, which calculates desired IOL power. Over the years, the difficulty has been in determining the desired correction with sufficient precision to eliminate the need for external corrective lenses. That problem still exists to a minor degree.

This same technique is now being developed, using phakic refractive IOLs to treat high levels of myopia and hyperopia. Clinical trials now are underway by several different manufacturers using a variety of approaches, including what is called the clear lens exchange (or clear lens extraction), the anterior chamber phakic lens implant, the posterior chamber phakic lens implant, and the iris-fixated contact lens implant.

Clear Lens Exchange

The clear lens extraction involves removal of the crystalline lens to replace it with an implant, as is sometimes done in cataract surgery. The crystalline lens has a clear outer capsule, which remains in place to support the new plastic lens. A significant drawback of this procedure for younger people is the loss of accommodation that results from removal of the crystalline lens.

If you remember from the third chapter, unlike the cornea, the crystalline lens has the ability to change its focusing power to adjust for near and far distance. This is called accommodation. As we age, we lose the ability to accommodate and eventually need eyeglasses for reading.

Although researchers are working on solutions to this problem, such as injecting liquid plastic or gel into the empty capsule to keep it flexible and placing the intraocular lens in front of the capsule, such techniques are some years away from clinical trials.

For older patients who already are presbyopic, the clear lens extraction might be an acceptable alternative. But most younger patients would prefer to maintain that ability to accommodate for as long as possible.

Another potentially serious drawback to clear lens extraction is the risk of retinal detachment resulting from the surgery. Highly myopic patients are at greater risk for other ocular problems, such as retinal tears and detachments, even when refractive surgery is not a consideration. Consequently, some refractive surgeons are reluctant to use this approach, particularly in highly myopic younger patients. However, other refractive surgeons are convinced that clear lens extraction has value, particularly for hyperopic patients.

An article in the ophthalmology professional journal *Eye World* asserts that "When it comes to hyperopic patients, however, most practitioners are more willing to try the clear lens procedure. John D. Hunkeler, M.D., former president of ASCRS [American Society of Cataract and Refractive Surgeons], in private practice in Kansas City and chairman of the department of ophthalmology at the University of Kansas School of Medicine, believes hyperopic patients with clear lenses are, in fact, the best candidates for the procedure and are likely to spur its popularity. 'Because of the shape of the hyperopic eye, it's less likely to develop retinal detachment,' Hunkeler said. 'Also, because it is a much smaller eye there is often not enough room for a phakic lens, especially in cases of extreme refractive error. The very place where space can be created is by removing the natural lens and putting in a synthetic one,' he said."

Anterior Chamber, Posterior Chamber, and Iris-Fixated IOLs

Three other phakic IOL implant techniques are in development, which leave the crystalline lens intact. One involves implanting the lens in the anterior chamber, the fluid-filled section in front of the pupil; another places the lens behind the pupil, in the posterior chamber; and the third clips and molds the implantable contact lens to the periphery of the iris, far from the margin of the pupil.

Anterior chamber lenses are made of polymethylen-emethacrylate (PMMA), while posterior lenses are made from soft materials such as collagen or hydrogel. Because these lenses are soft, they can be folded and inserted through a much smaller incision than those made of rigid plastic.

The rigid plastic lenses also have "arms" or "legs" that serve as anchors when the lenses are implanted. Notes Dr. Brint, "If not properly anchored, the lens can cause a blockage of the pupil, which leads to a condition called pupillary block glaucoma. This occurs when the implant blocks the natural flow of the aqueous fluid from behind the pupil through the pupil where it is then supposed to drain out the angle of the anterior chamber."

Glaucoma, as you read earlier, is a contraindication for refractive surgery. It is an asymptomatic condition often caused by other health problems such as diabetes. Pupillary block glaucoma is caused by the implant. Here's how. The eye continuously produces a fluid called aqueous humor, which drains out through the part of the eye called the "angle." When functioning normally, a balance is maintained and the intraocular pressure is normal. When fluid builds up because of a blockage or ocular disease, intraocular pressure rises and a patient is said to have glaucoma. Elevated intraocular pressure can lead to permanent damage to the optic nerve and loss of vision.

Also, it's possible for the anchor of the lenses to cause scarring in the angle, which could result in a blockage of the drain and also lead to glaucoma. Pupillary block glaucoma can be avoided by undergoing a procedure called an iridectomy several days before the lens implant. In this procedure the surgeon uses another type of laser to "blast" two small holes in the periphery of the iris, thereby creating another path through which fluid can drain. Anchors also can get tangled in the iris and distort the pupil, leading to a "cat's eye"–type pupil. This is not seen with iris-fixated or posterior chamber lenses.

There is some concern that if the IOL comes in contact with the crystalline lens, it will result in cataract formation. Explains Dr. Brint, "The posterior chamber phakic IOL was designed to avert this problem by vaulting over the normal lens. However, about a 5 percent incidence of cataract formation is being reported in large international studies with this posterior chamber lens. The cataracts either are caused by the lens itself or by the surgical maneuvers to place it behind the pupil."

A concern for all intraocular lenses is the potential damage to or loss of endothelial cells, the inner layer of cell lining on the inside of the cornea. The cornea is protected from swelling by these cells. Swelling is caused by excess fluid in tissue cells. The endothelial cells are capable of pumping fluids back out again; however, they do not regenerate. Once lost or damaged, they cannot perform the function of keeping the cornea stable. If cells are damaged during insertion, or if they are damaged when the eye is rubbed, maybe during sleep, bringing the IOL into contact with the back of the eye, the resulting endothelial cell loss could be significant. If progressive, it can cause corneal swelling and reduced vision.

Phakic IOLs and implantable contact lenses also have associated with them some of the complications and side effects associated with all refractive surgery, such as infection, glare, halos, under- or overcorrection, and fluctuating vision, among other things.

The advantages of implantable lenses is that they can treat very high degrees of refractive error; they are reversible, so if patients are unhappy with the results, they can have the implant removed; and visual recovery is rapid. However, phakic IOLs cannot be used to correct astigmatism, at least not yet. As with LASIK, there is minimal discomfort associated with the procedure. Most ophthalmic surgeons are very comfortable with phakic implants because they have years of experience with cataract surgery.

Surgeons are discovering that as satisfactory as LASIK is for most degrees of myopia and hyperopia, in the upper ranges (above -15.00 D) it is more difficult to achieve good results in the first or even second procedure. The ability to perform multiple enhancements to achieve good vision is restricted by the amount of corneal tissue available. If after a second or third procedure the patient is still not satisfied with his or her results, but there remains less than 250 microns of tissue, there is little recourse other than eyeglasses or contact lenses. Removing more tissue might weaken the eye and would leave no margin of error for age-related vision changes.

> *Surgeons are discovering that as satisfactory as LASIK is for most degrees of myopia and hyperopia, in the upper ranges (above -15.00 D) it is more difficult to achieve good results in the first or even second procedure.*

For this group of potential patients, the phakic implant or implantable contact lens might be the answer. Another option might be bioptics, where most of the refractive error is corrected with the phakic refractive IOL and the remaining small error and astigmatism, if present, is fine-tuned with LASIK.

Other Alternatives

There are many alternatives to laser vision correction, including contact lenses and eyeglasses. Some options do not involve surgery at all; others are accomplished with surgical techniques that, if performed by an inexperienced surgeon, can have disastrous results.

One nonsurgical alternative that you might have come across while researching refractive surgery is a technique called orthokeratology, which involves the use of contact lenses to change the curvature of the cornea over time. When removed, the cornea returns to its natural shape, but this can take days, weeks, and, rarely, months. In orthokeratology, specially designed contact lenses are inserted for specific periods of time to achieve the desired correction.

Most such contact lens programs require the patient to wear a series of lenses for varying lengths and then to wear a "retainer" pair of contacts for as often as one or two days a week to maintain the level of correction. The same risks associated with contact lens wear are associated with orthokeratology, and the correction is not permanent.

Some eye doctors believe that certain types of vision exercises can reduce refractive errors and prevent progression. If interested, you might do a Web search for Bates Therapy, or check your local library. Bates Therapy is based on relaxation and refocus techniques. Advocates and detractors are equally uncertain of the degree of its effectiveness.

There are a great many surgical approaches to the correction of refractive errors. Radial keratotomy (RK) is the most widely recognized. There also is astigmatic keratotomy (AK) for the correction of astigmatism and hexagonal keratotomy (HK) for the correction of low to moderate degrees of hyperopia. Anterior ciliary sclerotomy is an incisional procedure being studied for use in the treatment of presbyopia.

Keratophakia (KP) is yet another surgical correction for refractive errors at every level, including the most extreme. KP involves the creation of a corneal flap, as in LASIK, and the placement of a lens, either donor tissue or one made of hydrogel or some other biocompatible material, and then returning the flap to its original position.

Spectacles were invented in the thirteenth century, opening up a whole new world for people who could not see. Ever since, we've been trying to get rid of them. (See chapter 1 for the history of refractive surgery.) You can be sure that pioneers in ophthalmology will continue to develop and refine the technology and techniques that reduce or eliminate our dependence on corrective lenses. For the handful of people in the lens-wearing population who cannot benefit from currently available technology, there is reason to wait and reason to be optimistic.

For the rest of us, there couldn't be a better time to be myopic or hyperopic. For most people who depend on contact lenses or eyeglasses for good vision, the technology is as good as it needs to be to give you an excellent outcome right now.

10

Has the FDA Approved Laser Vision Correction?

It is a common misconception that the Food and Drug Administration (FDA) approves medical procedures. It does not. The FDA has no jurisdiction over the practice of medicine. It is, however, responsible for assessing and affirming the safety and effectiveness of products intended for use by physicians and other health-care professionals in the practice of medicine.

It may seem like a subtle distinction, but it is, in fact, a significant one. Drugs and devices that have been approved by the FDA for the treatment of a specific disorder can be sold in the United States for that purpose. An approved use is called an indication. Manufacturers include approved indications of the product in the labeling that must be affixed to a device or accompany a drug in its packaging. They also are allowed to promote such products for use in the indicated treatment but not for uses for which the product has not been approved.

However, the FDA does not monitor how doctors use those products in the delivery of patient care. It is not a medical policing agency. Doctors can use products for purposes other than that intended by the manufacturer, if they determine that use to be in the best interest of the patient and provided that use is based on sound medical judgment. This is called an off-label use or application.

> **The FDA does not monitor how doctors use those products in the delivery of patient care. It is not a medical policing agency.**

Standards of Care

Of course, this does not mean that doctors can do whatever they want or that there are no controls in place to screen out poorly trained or incompetent physicians and to protect the public's safety. There are a variety of mechanisms in place to ensure that doctors provide care based on commonly accepted standards.

The practice of medicine and physicians' behavior are the responsibility of state government. Every state in the United States has a medical board and many counties have medical review boards that set and monitor practice standards. Before doctors can practice medicine in any state, they must pass a licensing examination. Some states have reciprocity with other states, but not every state with every other state. For example, a doctor practicing medicine in the state of Virginia can obtain a license in the neighboring state of Maryland by filling out an application and paying an application fee.

States license doctors to practice, and they also discipline doctors for failure to exercise good medical judgment, up to and including stripping them of their license if it can be demonstrated that they are incompetent, impaired, or in violation of federal or state laws.

Professional medical associations provide peer oversight. Organizations such as the American Academy of Ophthalmology (AAO), the American Society of Cataract and Refractive Surgeons (ASCRS), and the International Society of Refractive Surgery (ISRS) recommend standards of care for the specialty or subspecialty within which its members practice, and they also outline ethical guidelines, including guidelines regarding marketing and promotional activities.

As mentioned in chapter 4, many doctors are certified by medical boards, which are independent, nonprofit organizations dedicated to improving the quality of care and to fostering excellence and encouraging continuous learning.

The American Board of Ophthalmology (ABO) will certify ophthalmologists after completing a comprehensive examination on general ophthalmology. As described on its Web site:

> The intent of the certification process of the ABO is to provide assurance to the public and to the medical profession that a certified physician has successfully completed an accredited course of education in ophthalmology and an evaluation, including an examination.
>
> The evaluation is designed to assess the knowledge, experience, and skills requisite to the delivery of high standards of quality patient care in ophthalmology. Periodic certificate renewal is meant to assure that members of the profession continue their education, keep current in information, and practice in a contemporary manner.
>
> The intent of the process is to set goals that will guide all members of the profession as they strive to keep up-to-date in knowledge and skills, and to practice competently.

In other words, a board-certified physician has demonstrated subject mastery in his or her area of expertise. Board certification is not required for a physician to receive a license to practice medicine but does evidence his or her level of skill and knowledge.

In addition, most health-care facilities establish guidelines for the use of medical devices and equipment by medical professionals. This is certainly true of laser vision correction centers. Although such corporations cannot tell a doctor how to practice medicine, they can request that physicians evidence appropriate education, licensure, certification, and competency before allowing them use of the facility. They also can refuse to permit use of the equipment to anyone failing to comply with those guidelines.

Off-Label Uses Lead to Medical Breakthroughs

Regarding off-label use of products, the presumption is that a medical doctor is qualified to make decisions about appropriate applications under specific conditions, based on his or her knowledge of the patient and the patient's diagnosis. Although doctors are free to use products for other than the intended purpose, they cannot promote the use of those products for other purposes. Therefore, doctors that performed LASIK as an off-label use were not allowed to promote the laser's use in that procedure, although they could promote the fact that they are LASIK-trained or have experience performing LASIK. This is very closely monitored by the FDA and by the Federal Trade Commission (FTC), which has jurisdiction over the marketing and promotional activities of all manufacturers.

As mentioned before, manufacturers cannot promote the use of their product for other than its approved indication. If found in violation of these restrictions, the company can be forced to stop production and shipment of the product until a government investigation has been completed. Physicians can be ordered to stop using a device if they are found to be promoting an off-label use, and the device can be seized if a government investigation finds doctors guilty of that offense.

The mere fact that a use is "off-label" is no cause for suspicion or concern. Prescribing drugs or using devices for other than the intended use has led to a number of important medical breakthroughs. Many currently available cancer treatments, for example, have come into widespread use as a result of physicians prescribing them for purposes other than that intended by the manufacturer. In July 1999, the *New England Journal of Medicine* released a study that demonstrated that combining a drug called Aldactone with standard medicines for heart failure—an unapproved use—cut deaths by 30 percent.

When drugs approved for one use are proved to be effective for other conditions, the manufacturer often will submit new data to the FDA and request that the product be given approval for use in the previously off-label treatment. This is sometimes referred to as an expanded indication. Once additional data has been reviewed and approval has been given, the manufacturer is then free to promote that product for use in the additional treatments.

For example, based on data gathered in studies conducted by private-practice physicians and by its own investigators, VISX Inc. and Summit Technologies submitted a premarket approval application (PMA) for the use of their excimer lasers in LASIK. In July 1999, the FDA Ophthalmic Device Advisory Panel recommended that the VISX Model C Star and Summit Technology's SVS Apex Plus workstation be approved for use in LASIK, and the FDA has since given its approval. Both manufacturers will be permitted to include LASIK as an indication on the labeling for those two devices. They also are able to promote that the lasers are approved for use in LASIK as a treatment for refractive errors. For all other excimer lasers currently marketed, LASIK is an off-label use.

That LASIK is considered an "off-label" use of the device does not mean that doctors are not permitted to perform LASIK. What it means is that the FDA and its advisory panel have not yet studied available data and determined that use of the laser in that procedure is reasonably safe and effective.

That the FDA advisory panel has not reviewed or made public its recommendation about a product's safety and effectiveness does not mean the data don't exist. Physicians around the world and in the United States have been compiling data on refractive surgery outcomes—including LASIK—for years. These data are widely shared at professional association meetings and in peer-reviewed medical journals (articles published in peer review journals are read and evaluated by subject experts other than the author). Refractive surgeons also freely share their own results with others and informally network with other surgeons to learn of new techniques that might improve results for all patients.

Physicians around the world
and in the United States
have been compiling data on refractive surgery
outcomes—including LASIK—for years.

Admittedly, the whole issue of FDA approval can be very confusing. In truth, almost since the excimer laser was first approved for use in PRK in October 1995, physicians also have used the device to perform LASIK. For example, as mentioned earlier, my co-author, Steve Brint, M.D., performed the first LASIK procedure on a sighted eye in the United States in June 1991 as part of an FDA-approved IDE. He has been performing it "off-label" since approval of the laser in October 1995 for use in PRK.

Because there was, and is, a great deal of confusion surrounding approved devices versus approved procedures, the FDA issued a letter to all U.S. ophthalmologists in 1996 regarding use of the excimer laser in refractive surgery. The letter stated that the excimer lasers manufactured by VISX Inc. and Summit Technology were approved for use in PRK but not for use in LASIK. However, the letter further stated that the decision by a licensed physician to perform LASIK was a "practice of medicine issue" and that the practice of medicine was outside the agency's jurisdiction. In practice of medicine issues, physicians are expected to use their medical judgment in determining what is in the best interests of their patients, given conventional standards of care.

As of this writing, the FDA has approved five excimer lasers for use in PRK to treat myopia, hyperopia, and astigmatism. Two have been approved by the FDA for use in LASIK. At least two physicians, Frederic Kremer, M.D., and George Waring, M.D., have received approval to use their independently constructed laser in performing LASIK to treat refractive errors, although Dr. Waring is not currently using this approved laser as he no longer considers it state of the art. Several other lasers are in various stages of clinical investigation prior to submission to the FDA of a premarketing approval application to make the lasers available commercially in the United States.

The Role of the FDA in Medical Device Approval

In 1976 the federal government passed the Medical Device Amendment to the Federal Food, Drug, and Cosmetic Act. This amendment required that all Class III medical equipment sold in the United States undergo a series of rigorous tests, called clinical trials or clinical investigations, to determine if a device being readied for commercial sale is safe and effective for use in humans or animals.

Medical devices fall into one of three classes, as determined by the level of risk subjects are exposed to when the product is used by a physician or other health-care provider. Cotton swabs and bandages are examples of Class I medical devices. The excimer laser is a Class III device because it emits radiation and because the potential for serious harm exists in its use. As you might surmise, Class III is the most stringent regulatory category. If a Class III device is unlike any current legally marketed device, its manufacturer must submit a premarket approval (PMA) application to the Center for Devices and Radiological Health (CDRH).

Devices manufactured and sold prior to 1976 were "grandfathered in," meaning companies did not have to go back and conduct performance tests or collect data to evidence safety and effectiveness.

The microkeratome is an example of a medical device that has not been approved for use in refractive surgery, as it was invented and sold prior to that year. Newer models do have to go through a review process but nothing like the exhaustive clinical trials imposed on excimer laser manufacturers. The microkeratome also is considered a cutting device and would in any case be held to less stringent regulatory controls than the excimer laser.

CDRH is the division of the FDA responsible for developing and implementing national programs to protect the public health in the fields of medical devices and radiological health. According to one of its own publications, "These programs are intended to assure the safety, effectiveness, and proper labeling of medical devices, to control unnecessary human exposure to potentially hazardous ionizing and non-ionizing radiation, and to assure the safe, efficacious use of such radiation."

Manufacturers of medical devices and products also must follow FDA regulatory guidelines established by the Food, Drug, and Cosmetic Act in the labeling of products, and must adhere to good manufacturing practices (GMP) requirements. These include disclosure regarding a manufacturer's organization and personnel, design practices and procedures, buildings and environmental control, device evaluation, distribution and installation, device and manufacturing records, complaint process, and quality assurance system audits. These are called general controls.

Class II devices also must conform to what are called special controls, which may include special labeling requirements, mandatory performance standards, patient registries, or postmarket surveillance.

By far the strictest regulatory practices are reserved for Class III devices, manufacturers of which must conform to all general and special controls and must also apply for marketing approval prior to selling the product in the United States.

Pre-Market Approval

PMA is the process of scientific and regulatory review enforced to ensure the safety and effectiveness of such devices. Manufacturers of Class III medical devices must conduct a series of tests called clinical trials, or clinical investigations, the results of which are submitted to the CDRH with the PMA application.

Contrary to popularly held beliefs, it is not the FDA that conducts clinical trials. It is the manufacturer's responsibility to recruit investigators from among the appropriate medical disciplines, to ensure that those investigators adhere to all applicable regulatory guidelines, and to collect, collate, and analyze clinical data received from investigators. In addition, the manufacturer must arrange for an independent review panel, called an institutional review board (IRB), to monitor the study. It is the responsibility of the IRB to ensure that the clinical trial is conducted in a manner that is medically and ethically sound.

Institutional Review Board

An institutional review board is precisely what it sounds like, a committee of individuals selected by an institution to review data collected by the organization to demonstrate the safety and effectiveness of a medical device or product. All university teaching hospitals have IRBs that meet regularly to review requests for approval to conduct research on human or animal subjects. Membership on these boards is by appointment and is for a specified period of time, usually two to three years. Any company or organization interested in conducting research may also establish its own IRB, but its composition must follow guidelines established by the National Institutes of Health.

> *Contrary to popularly held beliefs,*
> *it is not the FDA*
> *that conducts clinical trials.*
> *It is the manufacturer's responsibility to*
> *recruit investigators from*
> *among the appropriate*
> *medical disciplines and to ensure that*
> *those investigators adhere*
> *to all applicable regulatory guidelines.*

The primary function of the IRB is to ensure that studies conducted by a manufacturer, private-practice physician, or corporate entity conform to the ethical standards described in a report issued by the *National Commission for the Protection of Human Subjects of Biomedical and Behavioral Research.*

An IRB has authority to approve, require modifications to, or to disapprove research involving human or subjects. IRBs also have the authority to suspend or terminate approved research projects if they are in violation of the board's requirements or result in unexpected serious harm to study subjects.

IRB members must have the appropriate expertise and represent a cross-section of society regarding race, gender, and cultural or ethnic backgrounds to ensure sensitivity to the rights and values of human subjects. IRB members also must represent a variety of professions and must include those with scientific backgrounds and nonscientific backgrounds. Most IRBs have at least one person who is a member of the clergy.

Investigational Device Exemptions

For Class III devices, an IRB must approve study protocol prior to submitting an application to the FDA for an investigational device exemption (IDE). For anyone to use these devices in clinical trials, the FDA grants an IDE, which allows the manufacturer to sell and ship its device to an identified group of medical professionals who will participate in the trials as investigators.

Once a device has been approved for a specific indication (use) and is available for commercial sale and distribution, purchasers of those devices also can apply for an IDE to study unapproved uses. An example would be a private-practice physician who is interested in determining whether the excimer laser is safe and effective for refractive errors at levels higher than the current approved labeling permits. A company such as TLC, LCA, or Laser Vision Centers might also apply for an IDE for the same purpose.

Doing so has several advantages. One, it permits authorized investigators to use the device on a wider range of patients, albeit for a limited period of time. Another reason why users might apply for an IDE is to be "first on the block" to offer a new treatment once the laser is approved for that use.

An example of this would be the great many private-practice physicians and company-owned laser centers that applied for IDEs to study hyperopia prior to approval of the excimer laser for use in its treatment. Successful IDE applicants had the hyperopia software installed on their machines for purposes of the study. Once the laser was approved for that purpose, they were able to offer that treatment to all patients in the approved range, many months before competitors were able to arrange to have the software installed on their lasers.

Application Process for an IDE

An IDE application must specify the type of treatment to be studied, how many patients will be included in the study, and the duration of the study before the FDA will grant permission to undertake the study. The IDE application process is time-consuming, expensive, and labor-intensive. Briefly, here's how it works.

The sponsor of the device initially determines whether a device study presents a significant risk to human subjects. The proposed study is then submitted to an IRB for review. If the sponsor believes, and the IRB agrees, that a device does not pose significant risk, then a submission to the FDA for an IDE is not required. However, if the sponsor and the IRB determine that a device does pose risk to human subjects, then the sponsor must apply to the FDA for an IDE with the approval of an IRB.

In order to conduct a significant risk device study, a sponsor must submit an investigational plan, which includes such information as the study's:

- Purpose, including a description of the device and its intended use, and how long the study will take.

- Protocol, which is a description of the methodology to be used in the study and its scientific basis.
- Risk analysis, which describes risks to research patients and how those risks will be minimized, along with a description of the patient population to be included in the study.
- Device description.
- Monitoring procedures; how the sponsor will ensure that participating investigators adhere to the protocol and submit data.
- Labeling information.
- Informed consent document copies. Patients participating in a clinical study must sign a document affirming their knowledge that the procedure is investigational.
- IRB information, including all members of the review panel and their qualifications.
- Report of prior investigations, including a bibliography of all publications, whether negative or favorable, copies of significant publications, and a summary of other published information.
- List of all participating investigators, their qualifications, and the locations at which they will be collecting data.

The FDA can approve or reject an IDE application, even after an IRB has approved the study protocol and design. Rejection might be based on any number of grounds, including failure to comply with the IDE or other regulations, failure to supply requested information in a timely manner, or simply because the study is deemed to be too similar to other studies already in progress. Applicants for IDEs must receive in writing from the FDA word of approval or rejection. If rejected, the sponsor must be given the opportunity to appeal.

Reporting Requirements

If an IDE is approved, it is the responsibility of the study sponsor to ensure that all participants adhere to strict guidelines regarding device usage and outcome reporting requirements. A monitor must be selected whose responsibility it is to travel to each investigation site to ensure compliance and to report to the IRB and the FDA any study violations or unanticipated adverse events.

In LASIK, an anticipated adverse event would be the creation of a poor flap, requiring that the procedure be terminated for that day and the patient sent home to recover. An unanticipated adverse event would be a complication never before encountered during similar procedures.

Study sponsors are expected to keep meticulous records of every aspect of the study and be prepared to open those files to an investigator representing the FDA or the IRB at any time during the course of the study. The FDA also has the authority to conduct on-site investigations at any time and must be permitted "reasonable access at reasonable times."

Study Phases

Clinical trials for Class III devices are conducted in three phases. Phase I generally is conducted to study the effects of the device first on animals, then on donated cadaver tissue, and later on volunteer subjects. Phase I clinical trials for excimer lasers included the treatment of patients who were blind in one eye. This was done to help understand the effect of the device on living tissue, without unnecessarily endangering a patient's vision. In the Phase I clinical trials for VISX, a total of twenty-five patients were treated.

Phase II expands the study to a larger group of patients. This phase is designed to identify potential risks involving the device and safety hazards resulting from its use.

Generally speaking, the number of patients treated during this phase is quite small and close follow-up is required. Data gathered during this phase are submitted to the FDA for review and approval to expand the study for Phase III.

Phase III allows for treatment of a far greater number of patients, which gives the manufacturer the opportunity to learn about its device's effect on people of different ages, races, and sexes; and, in the case of the excimer laser, with varying degrees of refractive error. Patients in Phase III clinical trials also must be followed closely for a specified period of time. In excimer laser trials patients were followed for two years. Prior to the October 1995 approval of the Summit Excimed Excimer Laser, 1,600 eyes were treated and patients were followed for two years.

In every phase of the clinical trial investigators must adhere strictly to the submitted protocol. There can be no divergence from it unless the study sponsor submits an amendment. This can slow the study down or stop it altogether until the amendment is reviewed and approved. Consequently, there is little incentive for sponsors to change protocol in mid-stream, even if they learn that certain elements of the protocol could be adjusted to increase patients' comfort, for example, or to offer greater efficiencies of service.

Advisory Panels

Data gathered during clinical trials are submitted to the FDA for review by a group of independent experts, called an advisory panel. Data collected by excimer laser manufacturers are reviewed by members of the Ophthalmic Device Advisory Panel. Members of the panel are experts in the medical specialty in which the device will be used if approved. Many are affiliated with prestigious teaching hospitals. For example, the panel that recommended approval of PRK included Walter Stark, M.D., associated with Johns Hopkins University in Baltimore, Maryland. Its chairperson was R. Doyle Stulting, M.D., with Emory University Hospital in Atlanta, Georgia.

It is the job of the advisory panel to review submitted data to determine whether there is sufficient evidence that the device for which a PMA is pending is reasonably safe and effective. The panel makes its recommendation to the FDA after coming together in Open Session. In this session, members of the public are welcome to comment about the device in question based on their own experience or expertise. Frequently, a representative of the manufacturer will address the panel to argue favorably for approval of the device. Others who might address the panel would be physicians experienced in using the laser and even patients who have been treated by a physician using the laser.

> *It is the job of the advisory panel to review submitted data to determine whether there is sufficient evidence that the device for which a PMA is pending is reasonably safe and effective.*

Information about the time and place of these meetings is available from the FDA's office of public affairs, from the office of the CDRH, and on the FDA's Web site.

After the public hearing, the advisory panel makes its recommendation, which might be to reject the PMA based on lack of evidence or insufficient data; approve the PMA with conditions, such as further patient follow-up or additional outcome data; or a recommendation of approval without conditions.

That an advisory panel recommends approval does not guarantee that approval will be forthcoming, although the

FDA has a history of following those recommendations. Even an approval without conditions might generate an approval with conditions from the FDA. Prior to receipt of final approval, manufacturers receive from the FDA what is called a letter of approvability, which communicates the intent to approve and outlines any requirements to be met by the manufacturer before or after approval is granted.

Manufacturer Instructions

The FDA can and does impose on manufacturers of Class III devices any number of restrictions for use and requirements for distribution and assurance of safety. For example, when the excimer laser was approved, VISX and Summit were required to train doctors in its use, to certify and keep a record of each doctor trained on a specific laser, and to supply a patient education pamphlet to all doctors and facilities offering treatment with the excimer laser. Users were required to distribute those pamphlets to prospective patients prior to treatment.

Generally speaking, when treatment involves significant-risk devices, the FDA's instructions to the manufacturer about distribution and education will err on the conservative side. This is the genesis of many of the misconceptions about laser vision correction and why some have persisted for so long. When approval was granted, manufacturers were provided with guidelines that included instructing physicians to follow the same treatment protocol as was followed during the clinical investigation.

This is how the question of whether a patient should have laser vision correction on one eye at a time or both on the same day, known as simultaneous bilateral surgery, became an issue. During the trial period all study patients had one eye treated at a time, with a three-month interval between treatments. This was done to ensure the safety of study patients. In this way, if a patient had difficulty healing or experienced a sight-compromising complication, the fellow eye was still normal. It also gave surgeons the opportunity to study patients' healing response and to make adjustments to treatment of the fellow eye if indicated.

At the same time, refractive surgeons knew from extensive research and patient treatment in Europe, Canada, South America, and elsewhere that most patients vastly preferred simultaneous surgery. A sufficient number of patients worldwide had been treated to know that even though healing responses could differ from one eye to another in the same patient, this difference didn't necessarily require that eyes be treated one at a time.

Because the trial had been conducted one eye at a time, the manufacturers included that protocol in their surgeon training. Given the manufacturers' recommended treatment protocol, most malpractice insurance companies would not cover doctors performing laser vision correction unless they treated one eye at a time. Since then, this has changed, but the question of the advisability of bilateral surgery lingers in the laser vision correction lore.

So does the occurrence of postoperative pain. Early study patients did experience significant postsurgical pain because their eyes were patched for protection during healing. Today, a bandage contact lens is used and the incidence and severity of patient discomfort has been greatly reduced. Also, it took some time for doctors to determine the most effective postoperative treatment regimen. Since the introduction of anti-inflammatory eyedrops to control postoperative swelling and the introduction of the bandage contact lens as protection during epithelial regeneration, patient complaints of pain after PRK have greatly diminished. And with LASIK, pain has been all but eliminated. Many patients do experience a scratchiness that is described as similar to having grit in your eye or wearing your contact lenses way too long, but few describe the sensation as pain.

The approval status of LASIK arose from the restrictions imposed on manufacturers. For many months, there was no official recognition from laser manufacturers that LASIK existed as a treatment alternative or that lasers approved for use in PRK were being used for any other purpose.

Is the FDA Too Strict?

This is one of those questions to which there is no answer, although it's asked all the time in professional circles and in the general population. Other countries also have product-review procedures, many of them quite stringent, but doctors frequently have greater leeway in use of unapproved products, which is why so many breakthroughs in refractive surgery have occurred in Canada, South America, and Europe.

In the United States, a medical device cannot be approved until its manufacturers demonstrate that it is reasonably safe and effective. To do that, they must complete the clinical trials described earlier and submit the data for review. Data gathered by manufacturers elsewhere around the world, demonstrating that similar devices are safe and effective, are not considered in the approval process, even if the laser is of the same design and possibly produced by the manufacturer seeking approval in the United States.

Without our making a judgment about whether that's good or bad, it is time-consuming and expensive for the manufacturer and it delays the introduction of life-saving and/or life-enhancing treatments to the American public. Of course, it also prevents patients from being exposed to unnecessary risks before the technology and the technique are perfected.

Patients today being treated with the excimer laser can be certain that it has withstood the scrutiny of some of the world's most stringent manufacturing guidelines. And that can't be all bad!

Conclusion

If you've read through the entire book, then you probably know enough to make an informed choice about laser vision correction. Dr. Brint, Dr. Kennedy, and I have tried to include everything you could possibly want to know about refractive surgery and to anticipate your every question.

We've tried to curb our unbridled enthusiasm for the results of laser vision correction and present a realistic picture of what can and does happen before, during, and after the procedure. We hope we have succeeded and that you don't feel as if we're trying to "sell" you on the procedure. We're not. We know that many people are thrilled with their vision after surgery and that other patients out there are unhappy with their results. We also realize that some people just aren't interested in having their vision permanently corrected with a laser or anything else.

We've addressed some of the more outrageous myths floating in "cyberspace" these days. Since many people use the Internet as a primary source of health information, we searched the Net. We found a lot of information that was misleading, some of it dangerously so, and much that was just plain wrong. So, by all means, "surf the Net" but beware: Anyone can post anything and there is no one to verify its veracity. Don't believe everything you find on the Web, and if what you find raises questions, bring those questions to your doctor. If you're not satisfied with the doctor's answers, get a second opinion.

And don't believe everything you hear on television or radio, or read in newspapers and magazines. Sensationalism sells, and lots of times reporters get it wrong. Furthermore, there are so many doctors and laser vision centers competing for your procedure dollars that the din from advertising blitzes keeps growing louder. Health-care advertising is regulated, but lots of people try to push the envelope. Many claims being made simply aren't true. It's more important than ever that you do your homework. This book can help.

But you can't know, from reading this or any other book, what the experience will be like for you. You won't know how well you will be treated by the surgery center staff or if you will be among the small percentage of patients who experience a complication during surgery. And you can't know how quickly your vision will stabilize or if you will achieve your desired results.

You can't know for sure, but you can be pretty certain that your experience will be a positive one if you go into it with realistic expectations; if you truly understand that every single person heals differently and that the experiences of your sibling, coworker, physician, or friend may not be the same as yours.

Lots of people talk about the "miracle" of laser vision correction. You've heard of the WOW factor, which is the utter amazement some patients have when they wake up on the first day after surgery and their world is clear, maybe for the first time. But it also is possible that your vision won't be crystal clear right away, that you might have to undergo a second procedure, and that even then, you might have to wear glasses for some activities such as reading or night driving.

If your refractive error is low or moderate, your vision probably will be excellent after laser vision correction, very likely after only one procedure. But if your refractive error is high, you may require two procedures to achieve the desired correction, and it's possible that you may never be completely free of corrective lenses.

Before you say yes to surgery, make sure that all of your questions are answered to your satisfaction. When you sign the informed consent, you are effectively stating that you understand and accept the risks associated with refractive surgery. Be sure that you do. If the doctor minimizes the risks or tells you that the document is just written to scare you, walk away. Find a doctor who is comfortable talking about risk, confident in his or her ability to minimize those risks through surgical skill honed by experience, and prepared to deal with these rare complications should they occur.

If in this book we have helped to educate you about this potentially life-changing procedure, we've done our job and we're glad we could help. The two most important things to remember as you go through the decision-making process are these:

First, the decision to have laser vision correction is an extremely personal one. Don't let anyone talk you into or out of having the procedure. Only you know if it is right for you.

Second, have your surgery performed by the most experienced surgeon you can find in your area. When you watch promotional videos or visit facilities to view treatments, the surgeon may make it look easy, but it's not. That apparent ease comes with the experience gained by doing thousands of procedures. The decisions a surgeon makes before, during, and after surgery are made based on the results of those thousands of cases.

Remember, laser vision correction is for keeps, so see the best doctors and surgeons available.

Glossary of Terms

A

Ablation—The removal of tissue by vaporization with the excimer laser.

Accommodation—The ability of the crystalline lens to adjust the eye's focus from near to far and back again. As we age, the ability to accommodate decreases and we first need to hold reading material farther from our eyes, then must resort to wearing reading glasses.

Aniseikonia—A difference in the size of images created by each eye.

Anisometropia—A difference in refractive power between the two eyes of at least one diopter; for example, one eye is −2.0 and the fellow eye is −4.00.

Anterior Chamber—That space of the eye that is between the cornea and the iris, pupil and crystalline lens.

Anti-Inflammatory—A drug used to reduce swelling. Refractive surgery patients are given anti-inflammatory eyedrops to minimize swelling after the procedure.

Aphakia—The status of the eye when it no longer has its crystalline lens, usually as a result of cataract surgery, but this could also be the result of trauma to the eye. Until the lens is replaced with an artificial one, the eye is said to be aphakic.

Aqueous Humor—The fluid that fills the anterior chamber of the eye.

Argon—One of the gases used in the excimer laser to create the lasing effect.

Astigmatic Keratectomy (AK)—A surgical treatment for astigmatism that is achieved by making very small, deep, arc-shaped cuts in the cornea with a diamond-bladed knife, which "weakens" the power of the cornea that is too curved or "steep." AK weakens the cornea in the steeper axis but not the overall cornea, as does RK radial keratotomy.

Astigmatism—This results when the cornea is not round like a baseball, but oval, more like a football. People with astigmatism have blurry distance and near vision, and also sometimes have double vision, or "ghosting," because the light rays converge in two separate points rather than one.

Automated Lamellar Keratoplasty (ALK)—ALK is a refractive surgery technique involving the creation first of a corneal flap, just as in LASIK; then a second pass with the microkeratome removes a very small disc of corneal tissue. It is a mechanical way of removing corneal tissue that does not offer the precision of the excimer laser. Finally, the corneal flap is replaced.

Automatic Corneal Shaper—The microkeratome manufactured by Chiron Vision (now part of Bausch & Lomb Surgical); it is a cutting device used to create the corneal flap and was considered the "classic," or standard, for many years.

Autorefractor—An automated machine used to determine the degree of refractive error.

Axis—The direction of astigmatism is described by axis (horizontal or vertical) and by degree (from 0 degrees to 180 degrees); in other words, where the astigmatism is on the axis. Usually, the direction (axis) of the more curved part of the cornea is given (+ cylinder), but the same information may be obtained by giving the axis of the less curved (− cylinder).

B

Bandage Contact Lens—A low- or zero-powered soft contact lens given to PRK patients to shield the cornea until the epithelium regenerates, usually within three days. It is occasionally given after LASIK if the epithelial surface is rough at the end of the procedure from loosely adhering epithelium; it is also given to make the patient more comfortable and aid healing of the surface.

Best Corrected Visual Acuity (BCVA)—The best vision a person can achieve wearing corrective lenses such as contact lenses or eyeglasses.

C

Cannula—A syringe-like tool used to apply sterile saline solution to the cornea or under the flap during refractive surgery.

Cataract—A clouding of the crystalline lens, usually occurring in older people. Cataracts often are surgically removed and replaced with an artificial lens made of biocompatible soft or rigid plastic.

Central Islands—A complication of using the excimer laser in laser vision correction, in which the central part of the cornea receives less treatment than surrounding tissue, usually because fluid from the cornea tends to pool in the center and wet tissue is not as easily removed by the laser as dry tissue. Improvements in the laser software have greatly reduced the occurrence of this problem by adding extra energy to the central tissue removal process.

Co-Management—The practice of two doctors sharing treatment of a patient, based on each doctor's area of expertise.

Cones—Light-sensitive cells of the retina that are sensitive to color and function best in bright lights (rods are light-sensitive cells that are sensitive to black and white and are used mostly in dim light).

Contraindications—Pre-existing conditions that make it unwise to use certain medical products or pursue certain treatments. In refractive surgery, there are ocular and general health problems that can rule out surgery.

Cornea—The clear surface tissue of the eye through which light travels as it enters the eye. The cornea provides 70 percent of the eye's refractive or focusing power.

Corneal Topographer—A machine used to generate a four-color map of the corneal surface, usually indicating the high and low areas of the cornea and any astigmatism.

Crystalline Lens—The natural lens of the eye, located behind the pupil. Redirects the angle at which light travels through the eye, thus aiding the cornea in focusing light on the retina.

Cycloplegic Agents—Eyedrops used to temporarily paralyze the muscles of the eye to ensure an accurate refraction, thus preventing the patient from trying to accommodate or "over-focus," which would make the patient appear more myopic than he or she really is.

Cycloplegic Refraction—The measurement of your degree of refractive error, taken while the eye muscles are temporarily paralyzed from cycloplegic drops (usually the ones in the red bottles).

D

Decentration—A complication of excimer laser refractive surgery, resulting when the laser beam is not properly centered over the pupil. It usually can be corrected with a second procedure.

Dimer—A kind of gas; the argon and fluoride gases used to create the lasing effect in the excimer laser are dimers.

Diopter—Measurement of the degree to which light converges or diverges; equal to the reciprocal (reverse) of the focal length of a lens in meters. A 2-diopter lens brings parallel light rays to a focal point at half a meter. The term also describes lenses' refractive power.

Dry Eyes—A condition caused by deficient tear production or poor quality of the tears. Many people experience dry eyes as a side effect of refractive surgery. This condition is treated with artificial tears and occasionally with punctum plugs, which temporarily or permanently close the tear ducts that drain the tears away from the eyes. Dry eyes syndrome after laser vision correction usually subsides over time.

E

Emmetropes—People with no refractive error.

Emmetropic—The absence of any refractive error.

Endothelial cells—The cells that line the inner surface of the cornea, which pump fluids and remove them from the eye, preventing swelling of the cornea.

Enhancement—A second refractive procedure performed to help patients achieve the best possible vision, also referred to as a retreatment or "touch-up."

Epithelial Ingrowth—A complication of LASIK that occurs when epithelial cells migrate under the corneal flap.

Usually, this is treated by lifting the flap, scraping the cells away, and then repositioning the flap.

Epithelium—The top-most outer layer of corneal cells, usually a five-cell thick layer, which is removed in preparation for PRK or moved aside, along with a thin part of the underlying stroma in the form of a corneal flap, in preparation for performing LASIK. The tissue regenerates rapidly, usually within three days.

Excimer Laser—A medical device that concentrates a homogenous beam of ultraviolet light to remove tissue; used in the surgical treatment of myopia, hyperopia, and astigmatism.

F

Farsightedness—Also called hyperopia. It is the presence of a refractive error that makes it difficult to see near objects clearly and, when more severe or as the patient ages, far vision as well.

Federal Trade Commission (FTC)—U.S. government agency responsible for the oversight and regulation of advertising and promotional activities.

Fluence—The energy level of the beam of ultraviolet light created by the excimer laser. Insufficient or excessive energy can result in the removal of too much or too little tissue.

Fluoride—One of the two gases used in the excimer laser to create the lasing effect, which together constitute a dimer.

Focusing Power—The ability of a medium to direct light rays to the point of focus; also expressed as the medium's light-gathering power or speed.

Food and Drug Administration (FDA)—The U.S. government agency responsible for the regulation of manufacturers of medical products and devices.

Free Cap—A situation that may occur during LASIK, which results when the microkeratome cuts past the proposed hinge area rather than leaving a hinge. Experienced refractive surgeons consider this more a nuisance than a complication, as they are easily able to correctly replace the cap. This was the way LASIK was originally performed.

G

Glare—A usually transient side effect of laser vision correction that results in patients having some difficulty driving at night; typically associated with halos.

Glaucoma—An ocular health problem in which the pressure in the eye is elevated as a result of the aqueous fluid in the eye not draining out as rapidly as it is being produced. If left untreated, it can result in damage to the optic nerve and a permanent loss of vision.

H

Halos—A usually transient side effect of laser vision correction in which patients see rings of light around bright lights at night.

Haze—A usually transient side effect of laser vision correction, primarily PRK, in which the corneal surface has a cloudy appearance. Often the doctor can see the haze in a slit lamp examination, but the patient's vision is not affected. There are three grades of haze, the third being the most pronounced. If haze is present, it might affect vision, particularly at night.

Holmium Laser—A medical device used to treat hyperopia (farsightedness) with the application of heat in a spot pattern around the optical zone to shrink the collagen fibers in the cornea, creating a hard band that forces the corneal tissue up.

Hot Spots—The condition of the excimer laser when the beam is not homogenous and some part of the beam delivers more energy than the remainder. Laser technicians check for hot spots by testing the beam profile on a special plastic disc. Surgeons also can see when the laser beam is not delivering energy in a uniform pattern.

Hyperopia—Also called farsightedness. Hyperopia is caused by an eyeball that is too short or not curved enough to focus light properly on the retina. When light falls short of the retina, near objects are difficult to bring into focus.

I

Indication—The purpose for which a medical product or device has been approved by the Food and Drug Administration. PRK is an indication for which use of the excimer laser has been approved.

Intacs—Brand name of intrastromal corneal rings manufactured by KeraVision, which have been approved by the FDA for the treatment of low myopia (up to −3.00 D).

Intraocular Lens (IOL)—A lens made of soft or rigid plastic that is used to replace the crystalline lens, in the case of cataract surgery, or that is placed in front of it to improve its focusing power in the case of refractive phakic IOL surgery. IOLs used in this manner are more commonly known as intraocular contact lenses, which are still under FDA investigation in the United States.

Intraocular Pressure—The balance between the aqueous fluid produced and the amount drained. If there is too much fluid in the eye and it is blocked from draining, the result is a condition called glaucoma.

Intrastromal Corneal Ring—The generic name for tiny plastic arches implanted in the cornea via small incisions that are used to treat low degrees of myopia (up to -3.00 diopters).

Iris—Pigmented tissue that gives the eye its color. The iris lies behind the cornea and controls the amount of light entering the eye by varying the size of its opening, the pupil.

Irregular Astigmatism—A corneal surface that has "peaks" and "valleys," making it too uneven to correct with eyeglasses; however, rigid gas-permeable contact lenses often adequately correct the problem by creating a smooth surface.

K

Keratectomy—Removal of corneal tissue; see "Photorefractive Keratectomy (PRK)."

Kerato—A Greek word that means "cornea."

Keratoconus—A condition of the eye in which the cornea thins and becomes steeper, taking on a cone shape. It is usually considered a contraindication to refractive surgery.

Keratomileusis—Sculpting of the cornea; see "Laser in situ Keratomileusis (LASIK)."

Keratoplasty—Grafting of corneal tissue, as in Penetrating Keratoplasty (PK) or corneal transplant.

Keratotomy—Incision in the cornea; see "Radial Keratotomy (RK)" and "Astigmatic Keratotomy (AK)."

L

Laser—Acronym for light amplified by the stimulated emission of radiation.

Laser In Situ Keratomileusis (LASIK)—A surgical treatment for refractive errors that involves the creation of a corneal flap, application of the excimer laser to the inner layer of the cornea called the stroma, and replacement of the flap over the stroma.

Lasing Effect—The reaction created by the stimulation of elements such as gases, metals, or precious stones (rubies, sapphires) to create a laser beam. The excimer laser uses gases to create the lasing effect, which is then used to vaporize corneal tissue.

Lensometer—A machine that can "read" the prescription of an eyeglass lens.

M

Macula—The tiny area on the retina on which light rays fall for optimum visual acuity. The spot is $1/20$th of an inch in diameter.

Macular Degeneration—A sight-limiting ocular disease in which the macula deteriorates from bleeding (wet) or simple disintegration (dry), greatly reducing a person's vision.

Manifest Refraction—Measurement of refractive error taken without using cycloplegic agents. (See also "Cycloplegic Refraction.")

Microkeratome—A cutting instrument used to create the corneal flap in LASIK refractive surgery, of which Bausch & Lomb Surgical's Automated Corneal Shaper is currently the most widely used, though many newer models are now available in the market.

Micron—A unit of length equal to one-millionth of a meter.

Myopia—Also called nearsightedness; a condition caused by an eye that is too long or a cornea that has too much curve, causing light to fall in front of the retina and resulting in blurred distance vision.

Myopic Keratomileusis (MK)—A procedure in which the microkeratome was used to cut a layer of corneal tissue, which was then frozen, shaped on a cryolathe (device used to shape contact lenses), thawed, and then sutured back on the eye. With the introduction of the excimer laser and LASIK, MK is no longer performed.

N

Nomogram—A formula used to calculate how to program the excimer laser to achieve a desired correction. The number of laser pulses required to achieved a specific correction is affected by the temperature and humidity in the room where the laser is housed, as well as the altitude of the city. A surgeon's nomograms are developed over time as results are monitored and adjustments made.

O

Ocular—Pertaining to the eye.

Off-Label Use—A term used to describe the use of medical products or devices by physicians for other than the purpose intended by the manufacturer.

Ophthalmic Technician—A member of a doctor's staff trained in the use of ophthalmic diagnostic equipment, who assists the surgeon in the laser procedures.

Ophthalmologist—A medical doctor specializing in the comprehensive care of the eyes and vision. Although ophthalmologists have been trained to diagnose and treat medical problems of the eye as well as to prescribe glasses, typically, most primarily perform eye surgery.

Optic Nerve—The "connecting cord" of the eye that transmits electrical impulses to the brain for translation into images.

Optical Zone—The area of the cornea through which light passes and is bent (refracted) to achieve focus. Also, the term used to describe the diameter of the laser treatment.

Optometrist—Independent primary eye-care providers who examine, diagnose, treat, and manage diseases and disorders of the visual system, the eye, and associated structures, as well as diagnose related systemic conditions. Optometrists also prescribe glasses and contacts and may be trained to determine the best candidates for laser vision correction and provide expert postoperative care to laser patients.

Overcorrection—A complication of refractive surgery, resulting in a myopic (nearsighted) patient becoming hyperopic (farsighted) or the reverse. Overcorrections can be treated with a second procedure called an enhancement.

P

Pachymetry—A measurement of corneal thickness taken by ultrasonic probe.

PERK Study—A ten-year, multi-center study of radial keratotomy.

Phakia—The state of an eye that still has the natural crystalline lens.

Phoropter—An instrument used to determine the degree of refractive error. Lenses of varying focusing power are inserted in the device, into which a patient looks while the doctor asks, "Which is better, one or two?"

Photorefractive Keratectomy (PRK)—A refractive surgical technique in which the excimer laser is used to vaporize corneal tissue one-quarter of a micron at a time on the corneal surface, after the epithelial layer has been removed, usually by being scraped off. The epithelium regenerates in approximately three days.

Plano—A cornea with no refractive error.

Posterior Chamber—The "cavity" of the eye behind the crystalline lens and the wall or sclera of the eyeball, which is filled with the vitreous jelly.

Practice of Medicine Issues—A term used to refer to those decisions that are made by a physician and the patient, according to commonly accepted standards and that which is in the best interests of the patient.

Presbyopia—A condition caused by the loss of flexibility of the eye's crystalline lens, which results in the need to wear reading glasses, usually by the mid-40s but sometimes later. People with myopia can forestall the use of reading glasses by removing their distance lenses to read.

Ptosis—The name for any condition that causes the eyelid to droop.

Pupil—A circular opening in the middle of the iris that changes size to adjust the amount of light that enters the eye.

Pupilometer—An instrument used to measure pupil size.

R

Radial Keratotomy—A surgical treatment for myopia (nearsightedness), accomplished by cutting four to sixteen incisions to within 90 percent of the depth of the cornea with a diamond-bladed knife; advanced in the 1980s, first in Russia, then brought to the United States in 1986, and now has largely been abandoned for the more accurate treatment with the excimer laser, PRK or LASIK.

Refraction—The bending of light rays as they pass from one medium to another.

Refractive Error—The measurement of the degree to which light is bent, causing it to fall short of, behind, or at two different points on, the retina.

Refractive Surgery—Any surgical procedure that attempts to decrease a patient's refractive error; typically, this is accomplished by changing the shape of the cornea using a multitude of different procedures that are discussed in this text.

Regression—The partial loss of the correction achieved during refractive surgery.

Retina—The cell layers at the back of the eyes, which receive images and transmit them to the optic nerve.

Retreatment—A second refractive procedure that is performed to help a patient achieve the best possible results; also called an enhancement.

Rods—Light-sensitive cells of the retina that are sensitive to black and white and function best in dim light. (See also "Cones.")

S

Sands of the Sahara—A potentially serious complication of LASIK in which the cornea has the appearance of shifting, swirling sand. Also called diffuse lamellar keratitis, it is believed to be a noninfectious reaction and is treated with steroid eyedrops.

Slit Lamp—A high-powered microscope used to examine the eye.

Snellen Chart—The poster or projection in an eye doctor's office with a big E at the top and letters of decreasing size in a pyramid shape. It was named for Hermann Snellen, who first used it to determine a patient's visual acuity.

Striae—A complication of LASIK, in which the corneal flap has folds or wrinkles. They are treated by lifting the flap, smoothing out the wrinkles, and replacing the flap.

Stroma—The middle layer part of the cornea. The laser beam is applied to the inner stroma in LASIK, under the protective epithelial and outer stromal layer, to remove minute amounts of tissue to change the cornea's shape.

T

Tonomoter—A small, plastic, cone-shaped device used to measure the amount of pressure achieved prior to cutting the corneal flap with the microkeratome and also used to check the patient's intraocular pressure as part of a glaucoma check.

U

Uncorrected Visual Acuity (UCVA)—The best a person can see without corrective lenses.

Undercorrection—A complication of refractive surgery in which a patient falls short of the desired correction. It can usually be treated with a second procedure.

V

Visual Acuity—A measurement of how well a person can see. "Normal" vision is expressed as 20/20. A person with vision of 20/100 can see at 20 feet what a person with "normal" vision can see at 100 feet.

Vitreous Humor—The gel-like fluid in the main cavity of the eye behind the lens and pupil, the posterior chamber.

Appendix A:
History of Refractive Surgery

Many of us think of laser vision correction as something brand new because we are just now hearing about people who have had their vision corrected with the excimer laser. In fact, laser vision correction is just one more chapter in the long history of refractive surgery, which has been in development around the world for more than a century.

1880s

Advertisement for eyecup with spring-action mallet used to flatten surface; promises to "restore your eyesight and render spectacles useless."

Ophthalmologist L. J. Lans (the Netherlands) describes basic principles of keratotomy.

1939–1955

T. Sato and K. Akiyama (Japan) establish principles of transverse and radial keratotomy in rabbits and man.

Jose Ignacio Barraquer, M.D. (Colombia), refines lamellar keratoplasty for refractive procedures.

Barraquer uses the first microkeratome to cut a corneal disc.

Barraquer begins to use a more accurate microkeratome and invents the suction ring and guides for the microkeratome to travel along.

Ophthalmologist S. Fyordorov (Russia) perfects radial keratotomy.

Researcher Stuart Searles produces the first excimer laser action.

Ophthalmologist Richard Troutman introduces non-laser keratomileusis to the United States.

Barraquer organizes the first course on refractive surgery at the Instituto Barraquer De America.

1976–1986

Ophthalmologists around the world perfect keratomileusis techniques.

IBM researcher R. Srinivasan patents "photoetching" using the excimer laser.

Lasers become the subject of a study for use in the correction of refractive errors.

1983

Ophthalmologist Stephen Trokel (United States) experiments with the excimer laser for use in correction of refractive errors.

1983–1986

Ophthalmologist Luis Ruiz (Colombia) advances treatment of in situ keratomileusis (ALK) with new techniques.

Theodore Seiler, M.D. (Germany), uses the excimer laser to create "incisions" in blind eyes.

Ophthalmologist Leo Bores introduces in situ keratomileusis (ALK) to the United States.

Ophthalmologist Marquerite McDonald is the first to treat a refractive error with PRK on a normally sighted eye during clinical trials.

Ophthalmologist Lucio Buratto (Italy) uses the excimer laser on the corneal cap, which leads the way to LASIK.

Ophthalmologist Ioannis Pallikaris (Greece) advances the hinge technique.

Luis Ruiz, M.D., develops the automatic corneal shaper.

Co-author Stephen Brint performs the first LASIK in the United States in clinical trials.

1990–1996

Stephen Slade, M.D., Charles Casebeer, M.D., and Luis Ruiz, M.D., continue refining keratomileusis techniques, and the teaching of LASIK begins.

U.S. Food and Drug Administration approves the Summit Technology excimer laser for use in PRK.

U.S. Food and Drug Administration approves the VISX Inc. excimer laser for use in PRK.

As LASIK had already been performed internationally and in U.S. clinical trials, most refractive surgeons switched to LASIK as an off-label use of the excimer laser.

1999

FDA advisory panel recommends the labeling of excimer lasers manufactured by Summit and VISX for use in LASIK.

Appendix B:
Am I a Candidate?

General criteria to determine eligibility include:

At Least 18 Years of Age   Many surgeons recommend waiting until age 21; however, the lasers most widely available for LASIK were approved for age 18 and over. Internationally, LASIK is being done in children, especially when the prescription between the two eyes is very great and they can't wear contact lenses (see "Anisometropia"). LASIK can be easily redone at a later date in most cases (see "Enhancements"); thus, even when changes in the prescription are anticipated, more surgeons are tackling these situations. The conservative and traditional approach is to wait until there is stable refraction for one year, or fluctuation in prescription of no more than 0.50 D over a year's time. This kind of stability usually occurs in the early 20s.

Good General Health   People with the following problems should be carefully screened before having laser vision correction: uncontrolled diabetes; certain collagen vascular diseases; autoimmune diseases such as AIDS, although many AIDS patients have been successfully treated; rheumatoid arthritis; and scleroderma. Women who are pregnant or lactating should postpone refractive surgery until six months after the baby is weaned, as the prescription changes with the hormonal changes of pregnancy.

Good Ocular Health   People with the following ocular health problems should be carefully screened prior to having laser vision correction: glaucoma, diabetic retinopathy, retinal tears, keratoconus, cataracts, corneal infections, macular degeneration, severe dry eye, and very large pupils.

Refractive Errors   Laser vision correction treats refractive errors. It does not yet treat presbyopia, which is the loss of the ability to accommodate and results from aging, unless monovision is selected.

Realistic Expectations   Don't expect to throw away your glasses forever. Although the vast majority of patients can see without corrective lenses after refractive surgery, some still require lenses for certain tasks, such as reading or night driving.

Accept Associated Risks   There are common side effects, which are usually temporary but may be permanent, including such things as glare and halos around bright lights, sensitivity to light, dry eyes, fluctuations in vision, and some discomfort. These are all mild, transient, and generally resolved without physician intervention. The potential also exists for experiencing complications during the creation or the healing of the corneal flap, which might result in blurred vision, difficulty with night driving, double vision, ghosting, and loss of best-corrected visual acuity. Most complications are easily managed by an experienced physician but left untreated can cause serious vision problems.

Participate in Treatment   A successful laser vision correction outcome depends on a patient participating in his or her own treatment. This includes removing contact lenses prior to surgery as advised by the doctor; fixating on the light as directed by the surgeon; following all other physician instructions while in the laser room; following all postoperative instructions; and making and keeping all follow-up appointments.

LASIK Institute Guidelines

(The following can be found on the World Wide Web at www.lasikinstitute.org)

The LASIK Institute is a nonprofit educational organization dedicated to ensuring that prospective laser vision correction patients have the information they need to make an informed choice about refractive surgery.

The following questions appear on the Institute's Web site to help prospective patients think about the choice to be made. The answer to every question should be an emphatic Yes!

> Do you have a strong desire to be free of glasses?
>
> Do your glasses interfere with your job, sports, or daily activities?
>
> Do you clearly understand and accept the risks of surgery?
>
> Do you clearly understand that the effects of LASIK are permanent and do not wear off?
>
> Do you understand that refractive procedures require follow-up examinations at very specific intervals?
>
> Do you have time to attend these examinations?
>
> Are your expectations about refractive surgery realistic?

Also posted on the Institute's Web site is the following information about the position of the U.S. military regarding refractive surgery.

U.S. Army

Army Regulation 40-501 imposes some stipulations for soldiers and cadets who have the procedure. It does not permit someone who has had refractive surgery to come on active duty. If cadets get refractive surgery while at the Military Academy, they may not be commissioned upon graduation.

Moreover, soldiers who have had refractive surgery cannot go into training programs for aviation, airborne, Ranger, Special Forces, HALO (high altitude, low opening), marine diving, or combat diving. U.S. Army Link News states that the Army does not approve waivers. To the best of our knowledge, the Army has not reconsidered its position on refractive surgery since March 1997.

Air Force

Air Force Regulation 44-102, paragraph 1.27.1, states, "Performance of refractive surgery . . . is prohibited in all Air Force Medical Facilities, except by fellowship-trained corneal surgeons in direct support of the Wilford Hall Medical Center Ophthalmology Trained Program." Paragraph 1.27.3 further qualifies, "Active duty guard or reserve personnel who undergo refractive surgery must undergo a Medical Evaluation Board (MEB), and may be disqualified for continued duty."

Navy and Marines

The Navy is currently investigating the use of refractive surgeries with volunteers from their Special Forces. The Navy has published study results for PRK, but the military services are awaiting the results of the complete study of refractive surgeries before making a final proclamation. These results will not be released for several years.

According to the U.S. Naval Refractive Surgery Policy, the U.S. Navy and the Marines do accept waivers for refractive surgery. To be considered, military personnel must supply documentation of:

- Best spectacle-corrected visual acuity at 20/20 in both eyes postprocedure
- At least one year since date of the last surgery (or enhancement procedure)
- No significant visual side effects secondary to surgery affecting daily activities
- Stable refraction: defined as two refractions performed six months apart with no more than 0.50 diopters difference in spherical equivalence of either eye
- Preoperative refractive error not in excess of -8.00 diopters (spherical equivalent)

Applicants need to have a current eye exam and copies of their medical history. However, waivers are not considered for applicants to special duty communities (Aviation, Undersea, Diving, Special Warfare/SEAL) unless specifically approved by these communities' managers.

Nonetheless, one of the more interesting studies on PRK was done on Navy SEALS and Air Force Academy Cadets to determine not only visual acuity results but also effects of altitude, both above sea level and undersea. In this study the results were better with both the Summit and VISX lasers than the studies approved by the FDA in the general population.

U.S. Federal Aviation Administration Policy on LASIK

Accord to the Federal Air Surgeon's Medical Bulletin, Fall 1998, the FAA accepts LASIK for its pilots, as long as the FAA examining doctor finds "the postoperative condition has stabilized," pilots have "no significant adverse effects or complications," and their eyes meet the "appropriate vision standards" one to six months postoperatively.

The bulletin states that it is the pilot's responsibility to have his or her doctor send a copy of a report documenting outcomes to the Aeromedical Certification Division in Oklahoma City. This report will then become part of the pilot's permanent record.

Appendix C:
Frequently Asked Questions

If you are considering laser vision correction, then you probably have a growing list of questions. Below are answers to some of the most commonly asked questions.

Q. Can I go blind?

A. There have been no reported cases of permanent blindness resulting from refractive surgery. A very, very few people have had complications serious enough to require a corneal transplant, which, fortunately, is a routine operation for trained corneal surgeons, and donor corneal tissue, unlike many human organs, is not difficult to obtain.

Q. Will it hurt?

A. The procedure itself will be painless. Your eye will be anesthetized with eyedrops applied to its surface. It will be numb. Some people feel the slightest discomfort caused by the eyelid holder pressing against their eyelids, but it isn't usually described as painful. After the anesthesia wears off, your eyes will feel scratchy and uncomfortable. They may burn and tear excessively. This usually lasts only a few hours and you will feel much better if your eyes are closed—you usually want to take a nap anyway. For some weeks afterward your eyes may be dry. Frequent use of artificial tears will help.

Q. How long will the surgery take?

A. The procedure itself takes about ten minutes per eye, with the actual laser time being about thirty seconds, depending on your correction, however, you can expect to spend two to three hours at the laser facility in preparation for your surgery, for the surgery itself, and while you wait for the doctor to check your corneal flap prior to your being allowed to go home.

Q. How much does the surgery cost?

A. Fees vary by region, by surgeon, and by facility. Some charge more for LASIK than for PRK and more again for hyperopia and some forms of astigmatism. You can expect to pay around $2,000 per eye for PRK; $2,500 to $2,750 per eye for LASIK; and $2,750 to $3,000 for hyperopic LASIK. Once again, be wary of prices that seem too good to be true. There may be hidden charges such as the preliminary exam, topography exams, enhancements, and so forth.

Q. Will insurance pay any of the cost?

A. Probably not; most insurance companies do not cover the cost of the procedure as it is considered cosmetic surgery. There is no hard and fast rule, however, so you should check with your insurer. Growing numbers of vision plans now include refractive surgery along with eyeglasses and contact lenses as a reimbursable expense, and will pay toward laser vision correction whatever the plan pays toward other vision-care costs.

Q. Are payment plans available?

A. Yes, there are several options available. Most centers and many surgeons work with companies that offer financing at reasonable rates. Most facilities and many surgeons also accept major credit cards. If you have a flexible-spending plan at work, you can pay for your procedure with pre-tax dollars. Laser vision correction also is a deductible health expense on your federal taxes, and some people have been able to finance refractive surgery through a home equity loan. Your tax adviser is the person with whom you should discuss these options.

Q. Will I be able to throw away my glasses?

A. Maybe, but probably not forever. Younger patients with low to moderate refractive errors usually eliminate the need for corrective lenses at least until they reach their 40s; then they become presbyopic and need to wear reading glasses. Patients in the 40+ range often have to begin wearing reading glasses right after refractive surgery, unless they have elected for monovision. If you currently remove your lenses to read, there is a pretty good chance you will need reading glasses after surgery; you may even elect to not have surgery for this reason. Many patients with high refractive errors find that very thin corrective lenses for certain activities, such as night driving, are helpful. This depends entirely on how an individual patient heals.

Q. Is the surgery permanent?

A. Yes, the change to your cornea is a permanent change. Once tissue is removed, it can't be replaced. This does not mean that your vision will never change. It might. Some people become more myopic or hyperopic, as they get older. The laser can't adjust for naturally occurring, age-related vision changes, although experienced surgeons take age into consideration when determining desired correction.

Q. How quickly will I be able to go back to work?

A. Many people are back to work the day after the surgery; others need a day or two to feel comfortable driving or working at a computer for long periods of time. Each person heals at his or her own pace, but you can expect to feel more or less normal within one to three days. Hyperopic patients tend to recover sharp distance vision a little slower than myopic patients and may need to allow even a week or so off work if they elect to have both eyes done at the same sitting and sharp vision is mandatory.

Q. How soon after surgery will I see clearly?

A. That depends entirely on your healing response. Many people see clearly the day after surgery, although their vision continues to gain in clarity and stability for several weeks. For others, it takes several days for the postsurgery fuzziness to completely disappear. In any case it takes several months for your vision to finally "settle," to get that last 2 to 3 percent.

Q. Is PRK or LASIK approved by the Food and Drug Administration?

A. No, the FDA does not approve treatments or procedures; it approves products and devices. The FDA has jurisdiction over the manufacture of medical devices, not the practice of medicine. Six manufacturers of excimer lasers have received approval to sell lasers for use in PRK. Two have been approved for use in LASIK by the FDA.

Appendix D:
Tough Questions
to Ask Your Doctor

The Council for Refractive Surgery Quality Assurance (CRSQA) is a private, nonprofit educational organization established to make available to the public information about refractive surgery and surgeons who perform it. You might want to ask the following questions of a doctor (or a doctor's staff) whom you are considering for laser vision correction. Many, though not all, of these questions are extracted from the organization's Web site. Each is followed by an answer that falls within the range of what is usual and expected. Many of these questions appear elsewhere in this book. This questionnaire is by no means the only measure of a doctor's ability, but it is one more tool to help you make your decision about whether and with whom to have refractive surgery.

Q. How long have you been performing PRK and/or LASIK?
A. Not less than three years. The number of years the doctor has performed the surgery is not nearly as important as how many procedures the doctor has performed, but it is some indication of level of experience.

Q. How many PRK and LASIK procedures have you performed?
A. Not fewer than 500.

Q. How many PRK or LASIK procedures have you performed in the last twelve months?

A. Not less than 400. As with many activities, in refractive surgery practice won't ever make perfect, but it will ensure more consistent results. A doctor who performs hundreds of surgeries a month has fewer complications and more predictable results than a surgeon who only practices occasionally.

Q. Are you certified by the American Board of Ophthalmology?

A. The answer should be yes. Ophthalmologists can be certified by the American Board of Ophthalmology after taking a comprehensive examination in general ophthalmology. Certification is not required for a doctor to be licensed by the state, but it does evidence subject mastery.

Q. What percentage of refractive surgery patients treated by you achieve UCVA of 20/40 or better?

A. Anything above 90 percent is within a reasonable range. Many high-volume surgeons will have percentages that are even higher—95 to 98 percent.

Q. What percentage of refractive patients treated by you experience potentially serious complications, such as problems in the creation of the flap or healing problems such as epithelial ingrowth, Sands of the Sahara, and the like?

A. Most competent surgeons have a rate of serious complications in the range of less than 1 percent.

Q. What percentage of refractive patients treated by you experience minor complications such as glare, halos, or starbursts as long as six months after surgery?

A. A minor complications rate of 2 percent is within the normal range.

Q. Does your surgeon work with the same support staff or does it change from day to day?

A. Surgeons who routinely work with the same staff have fewer complications and better results than those who don't, as the entire team is involved in patient care.

Q. Have you ever had malpractice insurance coverage denied?

A. The answer should be no.

Q. Have you ever had your license to perform refractive surgeries revoked, suspended, or otherwise restricted?

A. The answer should be no.

Q. Is the excimer laser you perform refractive surgery with approved by the FDA?

A. The answer should be yes. If not, then you might want to ask the doctor if he or she has received an investigational device exemption (IDE) for the laser he or she is using. You should realize that you are participating in a study, which, after all, every early patient did initially to allow the lasers to be approved.

Q. How much will I have to pay if I need an enhancement to achieve the best possible outcome?

A. The answer should be nothing, within a defined period of time, usually a year. Most laser centers include retreatment in the global fee paid up front. If there is a charge, ask what the charge is for, such as an additional microkeratome blade or additional staff overhead.

Q. If my treatment is being co-managed by another doctor, will I have access to the surgeon and the surgeon's staff if I have questions or concerns?

A. The answer should be yes. The surgeon and the surgeon's staff should be available to answer questions or to provide follow-up care and management of minor or major complications if you deem it necessary or desirable.

Q. Will the doctor measure the size of my pupils?

A. The answer should be yes. This may be with a special instrument or by just examining the pupils in dim light. Some people have pupils that, when dilated in dim light, are larger than the treatment zones created by lasers in use today. Approval of lasers with wider treatment zones is coming; however, there is always the trade-off that larger treatment zones require deeper tissue removal and this is not always possible in high corrections or with thin corneas or enhancements in which the cornea has already been thinned.

Q. How many follow-up visits will I have and with which doctor?

A. Within twenty-four hours of your surgery, you probably will be seen by the surgeon or by someone on the surgeon's staff. Thereafter, if your surgery is being co-managed, you will see the co-managing doctor typically at one week, thirty days, ninety days, six months, and one year. Annual eye exams afterward are recommended and required by some laser centers companies that offer lifetime commitments. Additional follow-up visits may be necessary if you experience a complication.

Q. When will I be given a copy of the informed consent?

A. It's important that you read the document before the day of surgery. A week or so ahead of time is plenty. It's best if you read the document in the doctor's office or at the facility where you plan to have the surgery so you can have questions answered as they occur. If not, make sure to write them down or put question marks by the parts you don't understand so that these issues can be clarified to your satisfaction. Don't sign the informed consent until you are satisfied that you understand everything included. Don't be overly frightened by the informed consent, as it is intended to be an educational document and must by nature list almost every complication no matter how rarely it may occur. Don't be afraid to ask questions. They have all been asked before.

Q. Will you help me simulate monovision?
A. The doctor should be willing to fit you with contacts at no cost and give you at least two weeks in them to determine if monovision will work for you.

Q. Will you give me the names of patients who have been treated by you so that I might ask them about their experiences?
A. Most refractive surgeons maintain lists of patients who have agreed to speak to prospective patients about their experiences. You might also ask to speak with someone who shares your profession, your hobby, and your degree of refractive error. Your experience still won't be the same, but it will be closer than if you are in the moderately myopic range and the name you are given is a person who is hyperopic.

Q. Can I come to the laser facility to watch surgery performed?
A. Most laser facilities have viewing areas where patients, companions, and prospective patients can watch the procedure being performed. For most patients this is a very educational and calming experience, as they can see how easily and painlessly the procedure is performed and can talk with other patients right after their procedure.

Others, however, prefer to not see anything having to do with the eye. Do whatever makes you feel most comfortable.

Appendix E:
Fifty Steps to Improved Vision

Step-by-Step Summary of Laser Vision Correction

1. Learn your options, by researching vision correction alternatives.

   Books

   Laser centers: seminars; free evaluations; shop around and see where you feel comfortable

   Internet

2. Educate yourself about refractive surgery.

   Read

   Ask questions

   Talk to former patients

3. Decide whether laser vision correction is right for you.

   Do you have a strong desire to be less dependent on corrective lenses?

   Is this how you want to spend your disposable income?

4. Select a doctor or doctors to manage your treatment.

5. Discontinue contact lens wear prior to preoperative examination (LASIK Testing).

   Four weeks (and sometimes even longer) for gas-permeable or hard lenses

One to two weeks for soft lenses

Three days (seventy-two hours) prior to surger for all contact lenses

6. Determine your eligibility

Preoperative consultation

Questions about general health

Questions about ocular health, including any previous ocular surgery

Pre-operative examination, including:

Manifest refraction—without eyedrops, "Which is better, one or two?"

Cycloplegic refraction—with eye muscles temporarily paralyzed to prevent over-focusing and getting an incorrect refraction

Corneal topography—computer-generated map of the surface of your eye

Slit Lamp examination—check for surface irregularities and corneal clarity

Glaucoma

Pachymetry reading—determine thickness of your cornea

Pupilometer reading—determine size of dilated pupil in dim light

Fundus exam—looking at the retina primarily for holes or tears (more commonly seen in myopic patients) and to judge the health of the optic nerve

7. Discuss your decision with your significant other, family, and friends.

8. Ask questions of your doctor and his or her staff.

9. Make an appointment for laser vision correction.

10. Read and make notes of questions regarding the informed consent.

11. Travel to the laser center on the day of surgery.

12. Arrange to have a partner or companion available to drive you home.

13. Sign in at the center, fill out the paperwork, ask any additional questions, and sign the informed consent, which must be witnessed by one of the staff members.

14. Pay for the procedure.

15. The final corneal topography is taken.

16. Some visual exams may be repeated—a manifest refraction, for example—to ensure the accuracy of the numbers programmed into the laser.

17. Receive the postoperative instructions.

18. Greet the surgeon (or meet the surgeon for the first time and ask any additional questions regarding your particular case).

19. Discuss any last-minute concerns.

20. Receive your first set of eyedrops prior to surgery, antibiotic, anti-inflammatory, and numbing drops.

21. Put on a surgical bonnet if requested.

22. Enter the laser suite.

23. Lie down on the laser bed (it looks a lot like a dentist's chair).

24. The treated eye is prepared for surgery with anesthetic drops; possibly your eyelashes will be taped or surgical drape will be used.

25. The untreated eye is patched.

26. The technician tests the laser.

27. The surgeon ensures that the microkeratome is operating properly.

28. The surgeon and the technician double-check refractive numbers that will be programmed into the computer.

29. The surgeon places the suction ring on the eye to be treated.

30. The surgeon requests suction.

31. The surgeon tests corneal pressure with the tonometer, to see if pressure is adequate.

32. The surgeon squirts sterile saline or lubricating anesthetic solution on the cornea to lubricate the microkeratome pass.

33. The surgeon takes the microkeratome from the technician.

34. The surgeon places the gears in the track and guides the microkeratome across the cornea to create the protective flap.

35. Your vision will grow dim and likely go dark for a few seconds.

36. The surgeon lifts the flap to expose the inner corneal layer, called the stroma.

37. The surgeon instructs you to stare at the red or green blinking light.

38. The surgeon applies the excimer laser beam to the stroma (you will hear a clicking noise and either the surgeon or a technician will count down for you so you will always know how much more time you have). You may smell a slight burning odor even though this is only the corneal tissue being vaporized. There is minimal heat and, certainly, no burning occurs.

39. The laser stops.

40. The surgeon places the flap back over the stroma.

41. The surgeon squirts sterile saline solution under the flap to allow the flap to float back to its original position and to flush out any airborne debris (which rarely lands on the cornea while the flap is lifted).

42. The surgeon uses a Merocel sponge to smooth out the flap.

43. If it is a bilateral procedure, the treated eye is patched

44. Fellow eye is prepared for surgery.

45. The second procedure is completed.

46. You are escorted out of the laser suite and to the recovery area.

47. There you will rest quietly for ten to twenty minutes.

48. The technician or patient consultant will escort you to the examination room, where the surgeon or another doctor will ensure that your flaps are in place and the post-op instructions are clear.

49. Your companion will drive you home.

50. Take a nap. When you wake up, your vision probably will be blurry but you will begin to notice that you can see things you've never been able to see before without corrective lenses.

Appendix F:
Participating in Your Own Care

It cannot be stressed enough how important it is that patients participate in their own care. It can make the difference between an excellent outcome and a good or even poor outcome. Participating in your own care begins with the decision-making process and continues through a lifetime of good eye care. Do all that you can to ensure the best possible outcome from refractive surgery:

- Educate yourself about the procedure.
- Select a laser vision correction team that you feel comfortable with.
- Follow your doctor's instructions regarding contact lens wear.
- Arrive on time for your surgery appointment.
- Bring a companion with you who can drive you home.
- Fixate on the green or red light as instructed.
- Keep movement during surgery to a minimum.
- Go home and take a nap. Resting helps the healing process and makes you more comfortable during the first couple of hours when the burning and tearing are present.
- Use eyedrops as directed.

- Do not rub your eyes for the first month, then only very lightly after that.

- Wear sunglasses in daylight.

- Do not drive until your doctor gives you permission.

- Keep your first follow-up appointment on day one and every subsequent appointment, usually at one week, one month, three months, six months, one year, and every year thereafter, if participating in a lifetime commitment program.

- Do not wear eye makeup for one week.

- Do not use hot tubs, whirlpools, or swimming pools for one week.

- Avoid gardening and dusty environments for one week.

- Avoid contact sports such as football, basketball, rugby, or any similar activity that could result in injury to the eye for at least one month. Other physical activities such as jogging, weightlifting, and so forth, are fine after one day as long as you don't get sweat in your eyes and are tempted to rub them in this early period.

- Most important of all, use common sense. If you experience any unusual symptoms, such as pain that does not go away with use of Advil or Tylenol, excessive redness, itchiness, blurred vision, or swelling, call your doctor.

- If you have any concerns whatsoever, call your doctor. It's better to make an appointment and find out that what you're experiencing is perfectly normal, than it is to risk having a complication that could delay your recovery.

Appendix G:
Potential Complications of Refractive Surgery

What follows is a list of common side effects and potential complications that sometimes occur during or resulting from refractive surgery. Most side effects are transient, meaning they last only a few days and subside on their own. Some complications require medical attention. The incidence of complications in refractive surgery is very low, 1 to 2 percent for minor complications and 0.1 percent for more significant complications. For a better understanding of what each of the following terms means and how doctors treat these problems, read chapter 7.

Aniseikonia—A condition in which there is a difference in the size of the images created by the two eyes.

Anisometropia—A condition in which two eyes together have a significantly different refractive error and don't focus together in the same place.

Blindness—While there are no reported cases of permanent blindness resulting from laser vision correction, it is conceivably possible for blindness to result from an untreated complication of surgery. However, even complications that are left untreated, causing permanent damage to the cornea, can be treated by replacing the cornea with donor tissue. Corneal transplants are fairly routine procedures for specially trained corneal surgeons, and donor corneal tissue is not difficult to come by. There has been one reported case in which a severely myopic patient had retinal hemorrhages, which resulted in legal blindness, although it is unclear whether the LASIK had anything to do with this.

Decentered Ablation—This occurs when the excimer laser beam is not properly aligned with the pupil; it usually is treatable with a second procedure.

Dry Eyes—Dry eyes result when insufficient tears are produced to keep the cornea moist. Most people who have refractive surgery experience dry eyes for some period of time after the procedure, some for a few days, others for a month or more. The condition is treatable with the use of artificial tears, which can be purchased at any pharmacy, and occasionally with punctal plugs. Some patients experience somewhat dryer eyes permanently due to the new corneal shape not having as smooth a tear film as it originally did.

Flap Complications—During Surgery

Buttonhole—This results from a reduction in pressure during the microkeratome pass, creating an absence of tissue in the center of the flap, with a normal thickness in the periphery of the flap or a too-small circle of tissue rather than a corneal flap. It is treatable by replacing the defective buttonhole flap; waiting for the cornea to heal, usually within three months; and returning then for repeat surgery.

Free Cap—This results when the microkeratome pass fails to leave a hinge of corneal tissue. Usually, the procedure continues with the surgeon applying the excimer laser beam to the stroma and repositioning the properly realigned cap upon completion. This is how LASIK was originally performed; thus, for experienced surgeons it is considered a nuisance rather than a complication.

Thin Cap—This results when pressure is insufficient during the microkeratome pass. If the flap has adequate thickness, the procedure is performed as usual. If it is excessively thin, the procedure is stopped for that day, the cap is repositioned, and the patient is sent home to allow the eye to heal, usually within three months. The patient can then return for surgery.

Partial Cap—Same as previous.

Flap Complications—After Surgery

Epithelial Ingrowth—A condition in which cells from the outer layer of the cornea, called the epithelium, migrate under the corneal cap. It is treated by lifting the cap and removing—that is, scraping away—the cells from both the bed as well as the underside of the flap. If left untreated, the ingrowth can enlarge and can impair the quality of vision. In some cases there may be only slight, self-delimited ingrowth, which does no harm and is best left alone.

Striae—Folds or wrinkles in the corneal flap that cause the corneal surface to be irregular, reducing visual acuity and quality of vision. The problem is treated by lifting the corneal flap and smoothing out the wrinkles.

Glare—Discomfort in bright lights, resulting from an irregularity on the corneal surface or when the patient's pupil is larger than the treatment area. It can make night driving difficult. It is usually transient, lasting only a few days, but may be permanent, especially in people with very large pupils.

Haze—Haze exists when new collagen fibrils form proteins on the surface of the eye as the cornea attempts to "repair" itself after PRK, causing the cornea to appear cloudy. This is usually transient and often is undetectable by the patient. If it is pronounced and persistent, it can result in a reduction in the quality of vision. Haze virtually never occurs with LASIK.

Halos—Similar to glare; bright lights, such as headlights, appear to have a ring around them, making night driving somewhat difficult. Halos usually dissipate in a few days but can persist if there are irregularities on the corneal surface or the fully dilated pupil is larger than the treatment zone.

Infection—This occurs very rarely, as antibiotic eyedrops are instilled just before surgery, during surgery, and just after. PRK patients also apply antibiotic eyedrops on their own for several days after the procedure. Infection can result in scarring and a permanent reduction in vision. As previously mentioned, the incidence of infection with LASIK is less than it is for using extended-wear contact lenses.

Irregular Astigmatism—This results when the corneal surface heals in an irregular pattern. It can cause blurred vision for some period of time after surgery and sometimes results in a loss of best corrected visual acuity, meaning that the patient's vision cannot be corrected to the same level of visual acuity as before surgery.

Loss of Best Corrected Visual Acuity—This means that the eye cannot be corrected with glasses or soft contact lenses to see as well after surgery as it could be corrected to see prior to surgery. Often the loss of best corrected visual acuity means that a patient who could be corrected to 20/15 with gas-permeable lenses (which typically correct vision sharper than soft contacts) ends up with visual acuity of 20/20. However, some patients who could be corrected to 20/20 with corrective lenses can no longer be corrected to 20/20 after surgery.

Loss of Contrast Sensitivity—Some laser vision correction patients find that the quality of their vision, especially at night, is not as good after surgery as it was before surgery with their glasses or contacts, especially hard contacts. For example, postsurgery a patient might have difficulty reading in dim light or reading street signs that are not in sharply contrasting colors. This usually diminishes over time, but for some patients the change can be permanent.

Pain—Your eye is anesthetized during the procedure with eyedrops so you will not feel pain. Some people do say that the pressure of the eyelid holder against the eyelid is somewhat uncomfortable. After LASIK, many patients do feel some discomfort once the anesthetic eyedrops wear off. It is described as a scratchy, burning, or gritty feeling or as if you had worn your contacts too long. Post-PRK patients sometimes do experience significant discomfort, which usually can be managed with over-the-counter pain medications such as Advil or Tylenol.

Photophobia—Extreme sensitivity to light; it is experienced by most refractive surgery patients and generally subsides within a few days but can last a week or more. It is treatable by wearing sunglasses in daylight.

Ptosis—Drooping of the upper eyelid, caused by the lid holder stretching the muscles. This usually subsides on its own in a few days, and for PRK patients who use steroid eyedrops for several months, it usually goes away when the drops are discontinued.

Overcorrection—An outcome of refractive surgery whereby the outcome is greater than the desired correction. A myopic person who is overcorrected becomes hyperopic, and an overcorrected hyperope becomes myopic. Both are corrected with a second procedure; however, this usually improves with time so an enhancement should be delayed until the refraction is truly stable.

Sands of the Sahara—Also called diffuse interlamellar keratitis, it is the presence of inflammatory white blood cells of unknown origin that infiltrate under the corneal flap. They give the cornea the appearance of swirling, shifting sand. Certain doctors speculate that this is a toxic reaction of some kind. It is treated with cortisone-type steroidal eyedrops and sometimes by lifting the flap and removing the inflammatory cells, scraping away the debris.

Starbursting—A common side effect of refractive surgery, in which bright lights appear brighter and bigger than they are; similar to glare and halos.

Undercorrection—This results when the full desired correction is not achieved, meaning a myopic person would still have some degree of myopia and a hyperopic patient some degree of hyperopia. It is treated with a second procedure, called an enhancement, after the refraction is allowed to stabilize.

Appendix H:
Vision Correction Alternatives

Laser vision correction is the right choice for many people but not for everyone. It is important to know what your options are before making a final decision about refractive surgery.

Non-Surgical Options

Eyeglasses—By far the most common means by which people with refractive errors achieve good vision. Eyeglasses are relatively inexpensive and have associated with them only minimal risk of corneal damage if the lens breaks and scratches the surface of the eye. They can be uncomfortable, unsafe, or impractical when worn during many sports and other recreational activities. People with extremely high refractive error are not always able to achieve good vision with eyeglasses and find that their peripheral vision is compromised.

Contact Lenses—Due to changes in material used to make contact lenses, they have become much more comfortable and safer to wear in the past decade or so. Contact lenses can provide excellent vision, even for people with high refractive errors. They also can be inconvenient and can lead to dry eyes, corneal swelling, and warping of the cornea, and carry a higher risk of infection than does laser vision correction. Some people achieve better visual acuity with rigid gas-permeable lenses than would be possible with laser vision correction.

Rehabilitative Therapy—Some doctors believe that certain kinds of eye exercises can slow or stop the progression of refractive errors. For example, Bates Therapy is based on relaxation and refocusing techniques.

Orthokeratology—In this process, contact lenses are used to change the curvature of the cornea over time. The doctor prescribes a series of lenses to be worn for varying lengths of time to achieve the desired change. Orthokeratology takes time; there are limits to how successful the process can be and, because it involves wearing contact lenses, it carries the same risk of infection and other complications. Furthermore, because the cornea will return to its natural shape if left alone, "retainer" lenses must be worn periodically to maintain the desired correction.

Surgical Options

The LASIK Institute, a nonprofit, educational organization dedicated to informing the public about laser vision correction, outlines on its Web site the following surgical vision correction alternatives:

Radial Keratotomy (RK)—Is a refractive surgical alternative that involves making incisions in the cornea in a radial pattern. This procedure, refined by a Russian ophthalmologist in 1963, involves using a diamond scalpel blade to make usually four to eight tiny, spoke-like incisions in the periphery of the cornea. The incisions slightly weaken the peripheral cornea, causing it to bulge. This flattens the center of the cornea, thus reducing myopia.

Although currently a safer method than its predecessors, RK has its drawbacks. The resulting change in refractive error is felt to be less predictable because no one can control the way the incisions heal. As a result, RK may only reduce myopia, not completely eliminate it. Despite the surgery, RK patients may still need to wear glasses for distance. In addition, over time, RK can result in overcorrection, as was the case in 43 percent of patients studied over a ten-year period, as documented in the PERK (Prospective Evaluation of Radial Keratotomy) study. This is also known as progressive hyperopia.

Because of advances in laser technology, surgeons perform RK only on a very small numbers of patients.

Automated Lamellar Keratoplasty (ALK)—In ALK, the surgeon uses the microkeratome to separate a layer of the cornea and create a flap. The flap is then folded back and the microkeratome, rather than the laser, is used to mechanically remove a thin disc of corneal stroma below. The thickness and diameter of this disc determines the change in refractive error. The surgeon then places the flap back into position. This procedure can correct large amounts of myopia and hyperopia. However, the resultant change is not as predictable as with other procedures.

Photorefractive Keratectomy (PRK)—PRK was the next advance in refractive surgery (after RK). Performed worldwide to correct myopia, hyperopia, and astigmatism, PRK involves removing the epithelium, the surface layer of the cornea. Then a computer-controlled excimer laser reshapes the cornea of the affected eye.

Anesthetic drops in the eye ensure that the patient experiences as little discomfort as possible. The long-term visual results achieved are predictable and stable.

PRK has its drawbacks, too. Patients do experience discomfort for twenty-four to forty-eight hours while their epithelium regenerates. Some patients may have unstable vision for a few months. Others may experience varying degrees of corneal haze or cloudiness. Patients typically wear bandage contact lenses for pain reduction for a few days while the epithelial tissue regenerates and use postoperative eyedrops for anywhere from a few weeks to a few months.

Laser In Situ Keratomileusis (LASIK)—LASIK has been used for almost ten years to treat myopia, hyperopia, and astigmatism. It was first performed in the United States under clinical trials in 1991. In 1995, with the approval of PRK, the procedure became more widely available in the United States as an off-label use of the excimer laser.

In this procedure, the surgeon produces a hinged corneal flap composed of the outermost 20 to 25 percent of the cornea's thickness. The computer-controlled excimer laser then reshapes the underlying exposed cornea. The surgeon next puts the flap back into place. This minimizes discomfort and promotes rapid recovery.

LASIK resembles PRK, in that both procedures use the excimer laser to change the refractive error. However, because the surgeon creates the flap, LASIK preserves the epithelium and outermost stroma (the outermost 20 to 25 percent of the thickness of the cornea). As a result, the surfaces of the eyes treated with LASIK heal faster than those treated with PRK. Most patients achieve good vision the day following surgery. Furthermore, patients experience less discomfort.

LASIK requires more instrumentation than PRK, and additional surgical precision is necessary to handle the microkeratome.

Intrastromal Corneal Ring Segments (ICRS)—This procedure involves inserting usually two sections of a plastic ring into the mid-periphery of the stroma, which causes a slight stretching of the cornea and a subtle flattening of the corneal curvature. The change in the curvature varies with the thickness of the ring inserted. To insert the intrastromal ring, the surgeon must first create a small tunnel in the periphery of the cornea. Then the ring segments are inserted. This option to treat myopia has the theoretical advantage of reversibility.

KeraVision, maker of the Intacs brand of intrastromal corneal ring segments, recently received approval from the FDA for use of the rings in the treatment of low myopia (up to 3.00 diopters.

Phakic Refractive Intraocular Lens (IOL)—Used to treat a wide range of hyperopia and myopia, this procedure involves inserting an implant called an intraocular lens (IOL) into the eye's anterior chamber (the area in front of the pupil) or posterior chamber (the area between the iris and the normal [crystalline] lens). It is an advantage that this procedure has a long history with lens design and implantation technique for cataract surgery; however, using this procedure in patients without removal of their cataracts raises a number of concerns, and there is a risk of infection inside the eye. Further studies are needed to evaluate possible late-term complications.

The FDA has yet to approve any intraocular lens for use in the treatment of refractive errors.

Clear Lens Extraction—Used to treat a wide range of hyperopia and myopia, this procedure involves removing the eye's (crystalline) lens. The process is exactly the same as that of cataract surgery; however, in cataract surgery the lens is clouded, whereas in this surgery, the removed lens is clear. An advantage is that cataract surgery has been performed successfully for years and is a familiar procedure to many surgeons. There is more risk of infection inside the eye since this is an intraocular procedure. Also, clear lens extraction produces no accommodation (ability to see near without reading glasses) and possesses an increased risk of retinal detachment, especially in high myopia.

Appendix I:
Resources

Professional Associations

Each of these organizations offers information to the public on refractive surgery and refractive surgeons. Patient information is available on the Web site and by calling the organization.

American Academy of Ophthalmology
P.O. Box 7424
San Francisco, CA 94120–7424
(415) 561–8500
www.eyenet.org

American Board of Ophthalmology
111 Presidential Boulevard, Suite 421
Bala Cynwyd, PA 19004–1075
(610) 664–1175
(610) 664–6503
www.abop.org

American Optometric Association
243 N. Lindbergh Boulevard
St. Louis, MO 63141–7881
(314) 991–4100
www.aoa.org

American Society of Refractive Surgeons &
American Society of Ophthalmic Administrators
4000 Legato Road, Suite 850
Fairfax, VA 22033
(703) 591–2220
(703) 591–0614 (fax)
ascrs@ascrs.org
asoa@asoa.org

Joint Commission on Allied Health Personnel
    in Ophthalmology
2025 Woodlane Drive
St. Paul, MN 55125–2995
(651) 731–2944
(888) 284–3937
www.jcahpho@jcahpho.org

International Society of Refractive Surgery
1175 Springs Center, South Boulevard
Suite 152
Altamonte Springs, FL 32714
(407) 786–7446
(407) 786–7447 (fax)
www.isrs.org
www.locateaneyedoc.org

Excimer Laser Manufacturers

Autonomous Technologies
(division of Summit Technology)
520 N. Semoran Boulevard, Suite 180
Orlando, FL 32807
(407) 282–1262

Bausch & Lomb Surgical
(formerly Chiron Vision)
555 West Arrow Highway
Claremont, CA 91711
(800) 338–2020
(909) 399–1525 (fax)
www.blsurgical.com

LaserSight Technologies
3300 University Boulevard, Suite 140
Winter Park, FL 32792
(407) 678–9900
(888) 527–3235
www.lase.com

Nidek
47651 Westinghouse Drive
Freemont, CA 94539
(800) 223–9044
(510) 226–5750 (fax)
www.nidek.com

Summit Technology Inc.
21 Hickory Drive
Waltham, MA 02154
(617) 890–1234
www.summit.com

VISX Inc.
3400 Central Expressway
Santa Clara, CA 95051–0703
(800) 246–VISX
(408) 773–7055 (fax)
www.visx.com

Manufacturers of Other Refractive Technology

KeraVision, Inc.
(INTACS, implantable arcs)
47224 Mission Falls Court
Fremont, CA 94539–7820
(888) 846–8227
www.getintacs.com

Microkeratomes

Bausch & Lomb Surgical
(Automated Corneal Shaper, Hansatome, NuVita
   Phacic Refractive IOL)
555 West Arrow Highway
Claremont, VA 91711
(800) 338–2020
(909) 399–1525
www.blsurgical.com

Moria
15 rue Georges BESSE
f–92160 ANTONY FRANCE
33–1–46–74–46–74
33–1–46–74–46–70
www.lasikdiv@worldnet.fr

Refractive Surgery and Vision Correction Educational Organizations

Council for Refractive Surgery Quality Assurance
8543 Everglade Drive
Sacramento, CA 95826–3616
(816) 381–0769
www.usaeyes.org

The LASIK Institute
750 Washington Street
Box 450
Boston, MA 02111
(877) 405–2745 (Go LASIK)
(617) 636–0244 (Irene McLaughlin)
(617) 636–5754 (Laura Johnson)
www.lasikinstitute.org

The Optometric Refractive Surgery Society
2740 Carnegie Avenue
Cleveland, OH 44115
(216) 251–0969
(216) 251–0969 (fax)
www.orss.org

The Orthokeratology Institute
74 E. Main Street
Plainville, CT 06062
(860) 793–9613
(860) 747–6880
HBVC@aol.com

Government Agencies

These agencies have some responsibility for monitoring the manufacture and promotion of devices and equipment used in refractive surgery.

Food and Drug Administration
Center for Devices and Radiologic Health
Rockville, MD 20850
(800) FDA–1088
www.fda.gov

Federal Trade Commission
600 Pennsylvania Avenue, NW
Washington, DC 20580
(202) 326–2222
www.ftc.gov

Index

A

Accutane, 97

Activity restrictions following LVC, 145–146

Actors and actresses
as good candidates for laser vision correction, 41
having laser vision correction, list of, 25–26

Advertising
health-care, 242
for LVC, 183–186

Age
factored into vision correction, 2, 4, 160
vision changes occurring with, 265

AIDS as contraindication for refractive surgery, 96, 261

Air Force Regulation 44–102 about refractive surgery, 264

Akiyama, K., 253

Alternatives for vision correction, 18–20, 291–295

American Academy of Ophthalmology (AAO)
continuing education offerings of, 83
informed consent sample documents by, 126

peer oversight provided by, 223

American Board of Ophthalmology (ABO)
certification process of, 72, 223, 272
definition of ophthalmologist by, 72–73

American Optometric Association (AOA)
informed consent sample documents by, 126
licensing process of, 73

American Society of Cataract and Refractive Surgeons (ASCRS), 75
continuing education offerings of, 83
informed consent sample documents by, 126
peer oversight provided by, 223

American Society of Ophthalmic Administrators (ASOA), 75

Aniseikonia, 169, 285

Anisometropia, 169, 285

Ankerud, Eric, 202

Anterior basement membrane dystrophy, 103

Anterior chamber lenses, 215–218

Anterior ciliary sclerotomy, 219

M